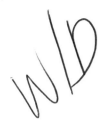

Cancer

Rehabilitation Medicine Quick Reference

Ralph M. Buschbacher, MD

Series Editor

Professor, Department of Physical Medicine and Rehabilitation
Indiana University School of Medicine
Indianapolis, Indiana

Spine

Andre N. Panagos

Spinal Cord Injury

Thomas N. Bryce

Traumatic Brain Injury

David X. Cifu and Deborah Caruso

Pediatrics

Maureen R. Nelson

Musculoskeletal, Sports, and Occupational Medicine

William Micheo

Geriatrics

Kevin M. Means and Patrick M. Kortebein

Cancer

Ki Y. Shin

Neuromuscular

Nathan D. Prahlow and John C. Kincaid

Cancer

Rehabilitation Medicine Quick Reference

Editor

Ki Y. Shin, MD

Associate Professor
Department of Palliative Care and Rehabilitation Medicine
The University of Texas MD Anderson Cancer Center
Houston, Texas

Associate Editors

Jack B. Fu, MD

Assistant Professor
Department of Palliative Care and Rehabilitation Medicine
The University of Texas MD Anderson Cancer Center
Houston, Texas

Ying Guo, MD, MS

Associate Professor
Department of Palliative Care and Rehabilitation Medicine
The University of Texas MD Anderson Cancer Center
Houston, Texas

Benedict Konzen, MD

Associate Professor
Department of Palliative Care and Rehabilitation Medicine
The University of Texas MD Anderson Cancer Center
Houston, Texas

Amy Ng, MD, MPH

Instructor
Department of Palliative Care and Rehabilitation Medicine
The University of Texas MD Anderson Cancer Center
Houston, Texas

Rajesh R. Yadav, MD

Associate Professor
Department of Palliative Care and Rehabilitation Medicine
The University of Texas MD Anderson Cancer Center
Houston, Texas

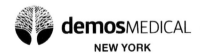

demosMEDICAL

NEW YORK

Visit our website at www.demosmedpub.com

ISBN: 9781936287048
e-book ISBN: 9781617050008

Acquisitions Editor: Beth Barry
Compositor: Exeter Premedia Services Private Ltd.

Medicine is an ever-changing science. Research and clinical experience are continually expanding our knowledge, in particular our understanding of proper treatment and drug therapy. The authors, editors, and publisher have made every effort to ensure that all information in this book is in accordance with the state of knowledge at the time of production of the book. Nevertheless, the authors, editors, and publisher are not responsible for errors or omissions or for any consequences from application of the information in this book and make no warranty, expressed or implied, with respect to the contents of the publication. Every reader should examine carefully the package inserts accompanying each drug and should carefully check whether the dosage schedules mentioned therein or the contraindications stated by the manufacturer differ from the statements made in this book. Such examination is particularly important with drugs that are either rarely used or have been newly released on the market.

Library of Congress Cataloging-in-Publication Data
Cancer: rehabilitation medicine quick reference / Ki Y. Shin, MD, associate professor, Department of Palliative Care and Rehabilitation Medicine, The University of Texas MD Anderson Cancer Center, Houston, Texas ; associate editors, Jack Fu, MD, assistant professor, Department of Palliative Care and Rehabilitation Medicine, The University of Texas MD Anderson Cancer Center, Houston, Texas, Ying Guo, MD, MS, associate professor, Department of Palliative Care and Rehabilitation Medicine, The University of Texas MD Anderson Cancer Center Houston, Texas, Benedict Konzen, MD, associate professor, Department of Palliative Care and Rehabilitation Medicine, The University of Texas MD Anderson Cancer Center, Houston, Texas, Amy Ng, MD, MPH, instructor, Department of Palliative Care and Rehabilitation Medicine, The University of Texas MD Anderson Cancer Center, Houston, Texas, Rajesh Yadav, MD, associate professor, Department of Palliative Care and Rehabilitation Medicine, The University of Texas MD Anderson Cancer Center, Houston, Texas.
    p. ; cm
  ISBN 978-1-936287-04-8—ISBN 978-1-61705-000-8 (ebook)
 1. Cancer—Patients—Rehabilitation—Handbooks, manuals, etc.   2. Oncology—Handbooks, manuals, etc.
 I. Shin, Ki Y., editor of compilation.
 RC262.C29163 2014
 616.99'4—dc23

        2013034862

Special discounts on bulk quantities of Demos Medical Publishing books are available to corporations, professional associations, pharmaceutical companies, health care organizations, and other qualifying groups. For details, please contact:

Special Sales Department
Demos Medical Publishing, LLC
11 West 42nd Street, 15th Floor
New York, NY 10036
Phone: 800-532-8663 or 212-683-0072
Fax: 212-941-7842
E-mail: specialsales@demosmedpub.com

Printed in the United States of America by Bradford and Bigelow.
13 14 15 16 17 / 5 4 3 2 1

This book is dedicated to our patients, whose courage, perseverance, and gratitude help inspire us to do what we do. Many of us have been touched by cancer, either in loved ones or as patients ourselves. All deserve the best possible care to help improve their survival. All deserve basic, thoughtful rehabilitation efforts to minimize the effects of the disease and its treatment. We have been fortunate to see and be part of an increased acceptance and growth in the field of cancer rehabilitation. We hope that the clinical information in these chapters will be used as a practical resource to help clinicians offer more rehabilitation care for their cancer patients.

Special thanks to Ms. Marilyn Lyles, whose significant efforts allowed for the completion of this project and to Dr. Theresa Gillis, who created the Rehabilitation Medicine program at the MD Anderson Cancer Center in Houston, Texas.

Contents

Series Foreword

The Rehabilitation Medicine Quick Reference (RMQR) series is dedicated to the busy clinician. While we all strive to keep up with the latest medical knowledge, there are many times when things come up in our daily practices that we need to look up. Even more important…look up quickly.

Those aren't the times to do a complete literature search, or to read a detailed chapter, or review an article. We just need to get a quick grasp of a topic that we may not see routinely, or just to refresh our memory. Sometimes a subject comes up that is outside our usual scope of practice, but that may still impact our care. It is for such moments that this series has been created.

Whether you need to quickly look up what a Tarlov cyst is, or you need to read about a neurorehabilitation complication or treatment, RMQR has you covered.

RMQR is designed to include the most common problems found in a busy practice, but also a lot of the less common ones as well.

I was extremely lucky to have been able to assemble an absolutely fantastic group of editors. They, in turn, have harnessed an excellent set of authors. So what we have in this series is, I hope and believe, a tremendous reference set to be used often in daily clinical practice. As series editor, I have, of course, been privy to these books before actual publication. I can tell you that I have already started to rely on them in my clinic—often. They have helped me become more efficient in practice.

Each chapter is organized into succinct facts, presented in a bullet point style. The chapters are set up in the same way throughout all of the volumes in the series, so once you get used to the format, it is incredibly easy to look things up.

And while the focus of the RMQR series is, of course, rehabilitation medicine, the clinical applications are much broader.

I hope that each reader grows to appreciate the RMQR series as much as I have. I congratulate a fine group of editors and authors on creating readable and useful texts.

Ralph M. Buschbacher, MD

Preface

Twenty years ago a perception of limited prognosis and limited benefit prevented many rehabilitation professionals from providing rehabilitation interventions for their cancer patients. Thankfully, since then we have seen and participated in a significant increase in the acceptance and availability of cancer rehabilitation care. As cancer patients are living longer, rehabilitation needs in this population will continue to increase. Rehabilitation clinicians can diagnose and treat the impairments associated with cancer. We can also help our oncology colleagues better understand and prioritize the functional aspects of our patients' quality of life.

Similar to the other volumes in the Rehabilitation Medicine Quick Reference Series, the scope of *Cancer* is very broad. Rehabilitation issues exist from prior to initial treatment all the way to palliative care. There are many different types of cancer, and their associated medical issues can be complex. Fortunately, many of the rehabilitation challenges presented by the various cancer types are universal and are common to other disease processes already familiar to rehabilitation clinicians. The purpose of this book is to provide a concise summary and treatment options for many of the issues a rehab clinician may encounter in clinical practice. The authors are experts in their fields and are associated with The University of Texas MD Anderson Cancer Center. I am very grateful for their assistance and participation in this project. The needs of our cancer patients will require the assistance of more cancer rehabilitation clinicians. We hope that this book will help you to meet some of those needs.

Ki Y. Shin, MD

Contributors

Etsuko Aoki, MD, PhD
Assistant Professor
Department of General Internal Medicine
The University of Texas MD Anderson Cancer Center
Houston, Texas

Annie Arteau, MD
Fellow
Department of Orthopedic Oncology
The University of Texas MD Anderson Cancer Center
Houston, Texas

Arash Asher, MD
Assistant Professor
Cedars-Sinai Medical Center
Los Angeles, California

Ahsan Azhar, MD, FACP
Fellow
Department of Palliative Care and Rehabilitation Medicine
The University of Texas MD Anderson Cancer Center
Houston, Texas

Walter Baile, MD
Professor
Department of Behavioral Science
The University of Texas MD Anderson Cancer Center
Houston, Texas

Diwakar Balachandran, MD
Associate Professor
Department of Pulmonary Medicine
The University of Texas MD Anderson Cancer Center
Houston, Texas

Lara Bashoura, MD
Associate Professor
Department of Pulmonary Medicine
The University of Texas MD Anderson Cancer Center
Houston, Texas

Karina Bouffard, MD
Clinical Pain Fellow
Department of Pain Medicine
The University of Texas MD Anderson Cancer Center
Houston, Texas

Sheryl R. Brandley, OTR
Senior Occupational Therapist
Department of Rehabilitation Services
The University of Texas MD Anderson Cancer Center
Houston, Texas

Brian M. Bruel, MD
Assistant Professor
Department of Pain Medicine
The University of Texas MD Anderson Cancer Center
Houston, Texas

Jennifer Camp, MD
Carolinas Rehabilitation
Charlotte, North Carolina

David W. Chang, MD
Professor
Department of Plastic Surgery
The University of Texas MD Anderson Cancer Center
Houston, Texas

Edward I. Chang, MD
Assistant Professor
Department of Plastic Surgery
The University of Texas MD Anderson Cancer Center
Houston, Texas

Eugene Kichung Chang, MD
Fellow
Department of Palliative Care and Rehabilitation Medicine
The University of Texas MD Anderson Cancer Center
Houston, Texas

Maxine De La Cruz, MD
Assistant Professor
Department of Palliative Care and Rehabilitation
    Medicine
The University of Texas MD Anderson Cancer Center
Houston, Texas

Rony Dev, DO
Assistant Professor
Department of Palliative Care and Rehabilitation Medicine
The University of Texas MD Anderson Cancer Center
Houston, Texas

Ahmed Elsayem, MD
Associate Professor
Department of Emergency Medicine
The University of Texas MD Anderson Cancer Center
Houston, Texas

Saadia A. Faiz, MD
Assistant Professor
Department of Pulmonary Medicine
The University of Texas MD Anderson Cancer Center
Houston, Texas

Carol Frankmann, MS, RD, CSO, LD, CNSC
Director, Clinical Nutrition
Department of Clinical Nutrition Administration
The University of Texas MD Anderson Cancer Center
Houston, Texas

Jack B. Fu, MD
Assistant Professor
Department of Palliative Care and Rehabilitation
   Medicine
The University of Texas MD Anderson Cancer Center
Houston, Texas

Ying Guo, MD, MS
Associate Professor
Department of Palliative Care and Rehabilitation Medicine
The University of Texas MD Anderson Cancer Center
Houston, Texas

Carolina Gutierrez, MD
Fellow
Department of Palliative Care and Rehabilitation Medicine
The University of Texas MD Anderson Cancer Center
Houston, Texas

Samir M. Haq, MD
Fellow in Oncologic Emergency Medicine
Department of Emergency Medicine
The University of Texas MD Anderson Cancer Center
Houston, Texas

Mary K. Hughes, MS, RN, CNS, CT
Advanced Practice Nurse
Department of Psychiatry
The University of Texas MD Anderson Cancer Center
Houston, Texas

David Hui, MD, MSc, FRCPC
Assistant Professor
Department of Palliative Care and Rehabilitation Medicine
The University of Texas MD Anderson Cancer Center
Houston, Texas

Carlos A. Jimenez, MD
Associate Professor
Department of Pulmonary Medicine
The University of Texas MD Anderson Cancer Center
Houston, Texas

Peter Kim, MD
Assistant Professor
Department of Cardiology
The University of Texas MD Anderson Cancer Center
Houston, Texas

Benedict Konzen, MD
Associate Professor
Department of Palliative Care and Rehabilitation Medicine
The University of Texas MD Anderson Cancer Center
Houston, Texas

J. Anthony Leachman, MA, BCC
Chaplain
Department of Chaplaincy and Pastoral Education
The University of Texas MD Anderson Cancer Center
Houston, Texas

Richard Lee, MD
Assistant Professor
Department of General Oncology
The University of Texas MD Anderson Cancer Center
Houston, Texas

Jan S. Lewin, PhD, BRS-S
Professor
Department of Head and Neck Surgery
The University of Texas MD Anderson Cancer Center
Houston, Texas

Valerae O. Lewis, MD
Associate Professor
Department of Orthopedic Oncology
The University of Texas MD Anderson Cancer Center
Houston, Texas

Gabriel Lopez, MD
Assistant Professor
Department of General Oncology
The University of Texas MD Anderson Cancer Center
Houston, Texas

Julie A. Moeller, PT, DPT
Physical Therapist
Department of Rehabilitation Services
The University of Texas MD Anderson Cancer Center
Houston, Texas

Megan Bale Nelson, MD
Assistant Professor
University of Louisville
Frazier Rehab Institute
Louisville, Kentucky

Amy Ng, MD, MPH
Instructor
Department of Palliative Care and Rehabilitation Medicine
The University of Texas MD Anderson Cancer Center
Houston, Texas

An Ngo, DO
Cancer Rehabilitation Fellow
Department of Palliative Care and Rehabilitation Medicine
The University of Texas MD Anderson Cancer Center
Houston, Texas

Susan Orillosa, MD
Clinical Pain Fellow
Department of Pain Medicine
The University of Texas MD Anderson Cancer Center
Houston, Texas

Karina Ramirez, MD
Fellow
Department of Palliative Care and Rehabilitation Medicine
The University of Texas MD Anderson Cancer Center
Houston, Texas

Suresh K. Reddy, MD, FFARCS
Professor
Department of Palliative Care and Rehabilitation Medicine
The University of Texas MD Anderson Cancer Center
Houston, Texas

Jennie L. Rexer, PhD, ABPP-CN
Assistant Professor
Department of Neuro-Oncology
The University of Texas MD Anderson Cancer Center
Houston, Texas

Kathie Rickman, DrPH, RN, CNS
Advanced Practice Nurse
Department of Psychiatry
The University of Texas MD Anderson Cancer Center
Houston, Texas

Janet Scheetz, PT
Physical Therapist
Department of Rehabilitation Services
The University of Texas MD Anderson Cancer Center
Houston, Texas

Vickie R. Shannon, MD
Professor
Department of Pulmonary Medicine
The University of Texas MD Anderson Cancer Center
Houston, Texas

Ki Y. Shin, MD
Associate Professor
Department of Palliative Care and Rehabilitation
Medicine
The University of Texas MD Anderson Cancer Center
Houston, Texas

Julio Silvestre, MD
Fellow
Department of Palliative Care and Rehabilitation Medicine
The University of Texas MD Anderson Cancer Center
Houston, Texas

Pamela Austin Sumler, LMT, NCTMB
Massage Therapist
Integrative Medicine Center
The University of Texas MD Anderson Cancer Center
Houston, Texas

Kimberson Tanco, MD
Assistant Professor
Department of Palliative Care and Rehabilitation
Medicine
The University of Texas MD Anderson Cancer Center
Houston, Texas

Alan Valentine, MD
Professor and Chair
Department of Psychiatry
The University of Texas MD Anderson Cancer Center
Houston, Texas

Khanh D. Vu, MD
Associate Professor
Department of General Internal Medicine
The University of Texas MD Anderson Cancer Center
Houston, Texas

Cynthia A. Worley, BSN, RN, CWOCN
Department of Nursing
The University of Texas MD Anderson Cancer Center
Houston, Texas

Rajesh R. Yadav, MD
Associate Professor
Department of Palliative Care and Rehabilitation Medicine
The University of Texas MD Anderson Cancer Center
Houston, Texas

Sriram Yennu, MD, MS
Assistant Professor
Department of Palliative Care and Rehabilitation Medicine
The University of Texas MD Anderson Cancer Center
Houston, Texas

Donna S. Zhukovsky, MD, FACP, FAAHPM
Professor
Department of Palliative Care and Rehabilitation Medicine
The University of Texas MD Anderson Cancer Center
Houston, Texas

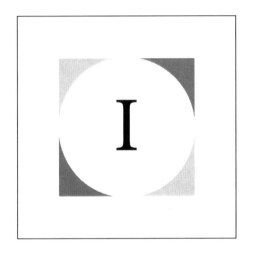

Background, Evaluation, and Interventions

Cancer Rehabilitation: Basic Ideas and Principles

Ki Y. Shin MD

Why Is Cancer Rehabilitation Necessary?

- Advances in the detection and treatment of cancer are allowing people with cancer to live longer. Survivors are frequently left with impairments that decrease quality of life.
- Rehabilitation strives to "make patients into people again" by addressing impairments, maximizing independence and function.
- Rehabilitation improves quality of life by helping to decrease the "burden of care" needed by cancer patients and their caregivers.
- Rehabilitation enhances function to help patients tolerate future treatments.

Much of the organized cancer rehabilitation efforts in the United States began in 1971 with support from President Nixon and his War on Cancer legislative actions. Significant early physician leaders included Drs Howard Rusk, John Healey, Melvin Samuels, Herbert Dietz, and Justus Lehman.

Stages of cancer rehabilitation described by Dietz include:

- Preventive rehabilitation efforts occur before cancer treatment begins and can help minimize functional decline from cancer treatment and its side effects.
- Restorative efforts occur after treatment to help bring function back to pretreatment levels.
- Supportive efforts in advanced cancer patients are directed at trying to maintain current levels of functioning.

- Palliative efforts are directed at symptom control and caregiver training at the end of life.

Problems in cancer patients amenable to rehabilitation efforts described by Lehman (see Table 1.1):

Table 1.1 Problems Amenable to Rehabilitation Efforts

Psychological/psychiatric impairments	Impaired nutrition
Generalized weakness	Lymphedema management
Impairments in activities of daily living, pain	Musculoskeletal difficulties
	Swallowing dysfunction
Impaired gait/ambulation	Impaired communication
Disposition/housing issues	Skin management
Neurologic impairments	
Vocational assessments	

- Many of these same issues exist in noncancer patients.
- Many rehabilitation professionals already have the education and clinical skills to assist cancer patients with a significant number of their problems.

Barriers to delivery of cancer rehabilitation described by Lehman include:

- Lack of identification of these patient problems by cancer clinicians
- Lack of appropriate referral by clinicians unfamiliar with the concept of rehabilitation

Factors affecting achievement of rehabilitation goals in the cancer patient described by Delisa (see Table 1.2):

Table 1.2 Factors Affecting Rehab Goals and Participation

Reduced life expectancy
Extensive comorbidity
Degree of pain interference
Dynamic lesions
Demands of current antineoplastic therapy
Desire to spend remaining time with loved ones

Logistics of Cancer Rehabilitation

- Cancer rehabilitation can be directed by a medical, surgical, or radiation oncologist; internist; neurologist; neurosurgeon; orthopedist; pain specialist; physiatrist and others.
- Cancer rehabilitation works much more efficiently with an interdisciplinary team (see Figure 1.1).
- Settings for cancer rehabilitation can include the home, outpatient clinic, outpatient gym, inpatient consultation, acute inpatient rehabilitation unit, skilled nursing facility, long-term acute care facility, and hospice.
- Common rehabilitation diagnoses can include aphasia, asthenia, deconditioning, hemiplegia, spinal cord injury, peripheral neuropathy, steroid myopathy, lymphedema, neurogenic bowel and bladder, limb amputation, limb dysfunction, and gait abnormality.

Helpful Hints

- Quality of life is subjectively defined by each individual, but commonly includes a sense of dignity. Maintaining function helps to maintain dignity.
- Cancer patients can have common rehabilitation problems.
- Educate oncologists to recognize the need and to refer their patients for rehabilitation interventions.
- Patient autonomy versus patient safety; cancer can force patients to choose one over the other, and it frequently becomes more about who can help you than how much you can help yourself.
- In the patient with advanced disease, further therapies may not make appreciable differences in function and may actually prevent patient activities by using up limited time and energy resources.
- Cancer rehabilitation will likely become as much about preventing disability (and cancer) as it is about restoring, supporting, and palliating cancer patients.

Suggested Readings

DeLisa JA. A history of cancer rehabilitation. *Cancer.* 2001;92:970–974.

Dietz JH. Adaptive rehabilitation of the cancer patient. *Curr Probl Cancer.* 1980 Nov;5(5):1–56.

Lehmann JF, DeLisa JA, Warren CG, et al. Cancer rehabilitation of need, development, and evaluation of a model of care. *Arch Phys Med Rehabil.* 1978 Sep;59(9):410–419.

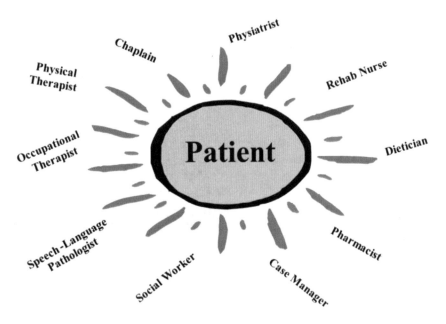

Figure 1.1 Interdiscplinary team.

Exercise

Arash Asher MD

Description

Cancer survivors face many challenges, including risk for recurrent disease, other chronic diseases, and persistent adverse effects on quality of life and physical functioning. Emerging evidence suggests that exercise can play a compelling role in mitigating these problems.

Goals of Exercise

- Improve function, aerobic capacity, strength, and flexibility
- Improve body image and quality of life
- Improve body composition, including decreasing body fat and improving lean muscle mass
- Potentially to reduce chance for recurrence or for a second primary cancer
- Improve anxiety related to cancer recurrence or in case of a second primary cancer
- Improve capacity to tolerate current or future cancer treatment
- Mitigate or prevent long-term effects of cancer treatment, such as osteoporosis and cardiovascular disease
- Improve cardiorespiratory, neurological, muscular, cognitive, and psychosocial outcomes

Pre-exercise Medical Assessments

- Evaluate for peripheral neuropathies and musculoskeletal morbidities due to treatment.
- Evaluate fracture risk for patients at risk, including those with metastatic bone disease and patients given hormonal treatment.
- Individuals with cardiac conditions (regardless of relationship to cancer) will need medical assessment of safety, including exercise stress testing.
- Breast cancer survivors should have shoulder mobility and lymphedema evaluation.
- Evaluate infection risk among the immunocompromised (i.e., avoid public gyms).

- Allow adequate time to heal after surgery (up to 8 weeks).
- Do not exercise individuals experiencing unexplained severe fatigue, severe anemia, or extreme ataxia.
- Caution for patients with an ostomy before participation in contact sports (risk of blow) and resistance training (risk of hernia).
- Thrombocytopenia: avoid high-impact exercises or contact sports. If severe, avoid all resistance training.

Exercise Prescription Goals and Guidelines

- Aerobic exercise: goal of up to 150 minutes of moderate-intensity exercise per week. The time frame to achieve this can vary depending on multiple factors including diagnosis, treatment, nutritional status, and so forth.
- Strength training: goal of 2 to 3 weekly sessions
- Flexibility: stretch major muscle groups several days per week

Exercise Challenges and Precautions

- Changes in swelling/lymphedema should result in reductions or avoidance of upper body exercise until the patient is evaluated.
- Patients with lymphedema should wear a well-fitted compression garment during exercise.
- If metastatic disease is present in bone (especially weight bearing), an exercise regimen will need modifications and increased supervision.
- Exercise tolerance of cancer patients during treatment may vary from session to session.
- Exercise adherence is a major challenge and supportive counseling should be provided.

Mortality Benefits of Exercise for Cancer Patients

- Exercise *may* extend survival for some cancer patients, including those with breast and colon cancer.
- Other cancers need more research.

Helpful Hints

- If peripheral neuropathy is present, a stationary recumbent bike may be preferable over weight-bearing exercise.
- Add pelvic floor exercises for those who undergo radical prostatectomy.
- Use resistance training and aerobic exercise in bone marrow transplant patients.
- Resistance training can be performed safely by breast cancer survivors with and at risk for lymphedema; avoid fatiguing exercises.
- Water-based exercises may be very useful, especially for patients at risk for falls.

Useful Consultants

- Physiatrist
- Exercise physiologist
- Physical therapist
- Fitness trainers experienced with cancer survivors

Summary/Conclusions

- Exercise training is generally very safe during and after cancer treatments and can result in improvements in physical functioning, quality of life, and cancer-related fatigue.

Suggested Readings

American College of Sports Medicine. *Guidelines for Exercise Testing and Prescription.* 8th ed. Philadelphia, PA: Lippincott, Wilkins, and Williams; 2009.

Schmitz K, Ahmed RL, Troxel A, et al. Weight lifting in women with breast-cancer-related lymphedema. *N Engl J Med.* 2009;361:664–673.

Schmitz KH, Courneya KS, Matthews C, et al. American College of Sports Medicine roundtable on exercise guidelines for cancer survivors. *Med Sci Sports Exer.* 42:1409–1426. doi: 10.1249/MSS.0b013e3181e0c112

Occupational Therapy

Sheryl R. Brandley OTR

Description

Supporting health and participation in life through engagement in occupation describes the domain in its fullest sense. Within this diverse field, the defining contribution of occupational therapy is the application of core values, knowledge, and skills to assist patients to engage in everyday activities or occupations that they want and need to do in a manner that supports health and participation.

Because occupational therapy practitioners view patients holistically, they consider factors that involve the values, beliefs, and spirituality; body functions; and body structures.

The unique contribution of occupational therapy is to prepare patients to go home safely or to assist them to move to the next level of care. That level of care can range from a skilled nursing facility, long-term acute care, or home with family.

Owing to the numerous types of cancer, occupational therapy treatment focuses on the symptoms that decrease engagement in activities of daily living (ADLs)/instrumental activities of daily living (IADLs). Some of these symptoms include: malaise and fatigue, muscle weakness, lack of coordination, decreased memory skills, edema, impaired cognition, and pain.

Examination

- ADL functions—patients are assessed on current functional performance with ADLs through the use of functional independence measure scores and other standardized deficit-specific assessments. Occupational profiles assure client-centered goals and treatment plan.
- Cognitive function screening—assessment of memory, attention span, decision-making skills, executive decisions, problem solving, and so forth
- Musculoskeletal function—testing of range of motion, strength, posture, tone, and joint mobility
- Neuromuscular function—testing of balance, coordination, reflexes, hearing, and vision
- Cardiovascular/pulmonary function—assessment of edema, endurance during the performance of ADL tasks
- Seating and mobility

Factors Affecting Therapy

- Difficulty with mobility due to IV poles with multiple medications
- Plastic surgery restrictions may require the use of assistive or seating devices.
- Skin fragility due to weight loss, low platelets, or increased edema during cancer treatment
- Increased fatigue from cancer treatment or disease process
- Infections may decrease stamina for the performance of ADLs.
- Decreased safety and cognition due to medications that may affect balance and problem solving
- Difficulty performing ADLs for orthopedic patients due to surgical pain and wounds
- Decreased standing tolerance or balance while on chemotherapy or other medications
- Impaired sensation in hands due to chemotherapy, which can affect grip during ADLs
- Impaired vision due to cancer or cancer-related treatment
- Laminectomy and sternal precautions that limit certain postures during the performance of ADLs
- Lack of volition due to loss of routines and roles
- Chemotherapy or infections that cause mouth sores or bleeding gums may affect feeding ADLs.
- Chemotherapy treatments that produce nausea, vomiting, and loose stools may affect patient participation in treatment.
- Radiation, which may cause hypersensitivity of the skin during the performance of ADLs

Treatment

- Improve performance of ADLs and IADLs
- Education and training through the use of assistive devices or durable medical equipment

- Education and training of caregivers
- Therapeutic exercises and activities
- Home exercise programs
- Splinting and bracing
- Fatigue and fall prevention
- Neuromuscular reeducation
- Modalities
- Wheelchair training and management
- Cognitive retraining/adaptation
- Pain management
- Community reintegration

Helpful Hints
- Infection control is a priority owing to the impaired immune system of many of these patients.
- Fatigue in cancer patients requires special management techniques.
- The family is very important in the rehabilitation training process.

Suggested Reading
American Occupational Therapy Association. *Occupational Therapy Practice Framework: Domain & Process.* 2nd ed. Bethesda, MA: AOTA Press; 2008.

I: Background, Evaluation, and Interventions

Performance Measures

Jack B. Fu MD

Description

A variety of performance measures are used in the oncologic setting. The Functional Independence Measure (FIM; Figure 4.1) is the mostly widely used clinically among physiatrists. It is useful to become familiar with various performance scales, in particular the Karnofsky (see Table 4.1) and the ECOG (Eastern Cooperative Oncology Group; see Table 4.2). Oncologists will use these scales when discussing their patients. The scales are mainly used by oncologists for prognostic information and in the decision process for cancer treatments.

Karnofsky Performance Scale

The Karnofsky Performance Scale Index allows patients to be classified as per their functional impairment. This can be used to compare effectiveness of different therapies and to assess the prognosis in individual patients. The lower the Karnofsky score, the worse the survival for most serious illnesses.

Table 4.1 Karnofsky Performance Status Scale Definitions Rating (%) Criteria

Able to carry on normal activity and to work; no special care needed	100	Normal, no complaints; no evidence of disease
	90	Able to carry on normal activity; minor signs or symptoms of disease
	80	Normal activity with effort; some signs or symptoms of disease
Unable to work; able to live at home and care for most personal needs; varying amount of assistance needed	70	Cares for self; unable to carry on normal activity or to do active work
	60	Requires occasional assistance, but is able to care for most of his or her personal needs
	50	Requires considerable assistance and frequent medical care
Unable to care for self; requires equivalent of institutional or hospital care; disease may be progressing rapidly	40	Disabled; requires special care and assistance
	30	Severely disabled; hospital admission is indicated although death not imminent
	20	Very sick; hospital admission necessary; active supportive treatment necessary
	10	Moribund; fatal processes progressing rapidly
	0	Dead

ECOG Performance Scale

Table 4.2 ECOG Performance Status

Grade	ECOG
0	Fully active, able to carry on all predisease performance without restriction
1	Restricted in physically strenuous activity but ambulatory and able to carry out work of a light or sedentary nature, for example, light housework, office work
2	Ambulatory and capable of all self-care but unable to carry out any work activities. Up and about more than 50% of waking hours
3	Capable of only limited self-care, confined to bed or chair more than 50% of waking hours
4	Completely disabled. Cannot carry on any self-care. Totally confined to bed or chair
5	Dead

Source: Oken et al. (1982).

LEVELS		
	7 Complete Independence (timely, safely) 6 Modified Independence (device)	**NO HELPER**
	Modified Dependence 5 Supervision (subject = 100%) 4 Minimal Assistance (subject = 75%+) 3 Moderate Assistance (subject = 50%+) **Complete Dependence** 2 Maximal Assistance (subject = 25%+) 1 Total Assistance (subject = less than 25%)	**HELPER**

	ADMISSION	DISCHARGE	FOLLOW-UP
Self-Care			
A. Eating			
B. Grooming			
C. Bathing			
D. Dressing - Upper Body			
E. Dressing - Lower Body			
F. Toileting			
Sphincter Control			
G. Bladder Management			
H. Bowel Management			
Transfers			
I. Bed, Chair, Wheelchair			
J. Toilet			
K. Tub, Shower			
Locomotion			
L. Walk/Wheelchair	W Walk C Wheelchair B Both	W Walk C Wheelchair B Both	W Walk C Wheelchair B Both
M. Stairs			
Motor Subtotal Score			
Communication			
N. Comprehension	A Auditory V Visual B Both	A Auditory V Visual B Both	A Auditory V Visual B Both
O. Expression	A Auditory V Visual B Both	A Auditory V Visual B Both	A Auditory V Visual B Both
Social Cognition			
P. Social Interaction			
Q. Problem Solving			
R. Memory			
Cognitive Subtotal Score			
TOTAL FIM™ SCORE			

NOTE: Leave no blanks. Enter 1 if patient is not testable due to risk.

Figure 4.1 FIM instrument.

Get Up and Go Test

The Get Up and Go test is used to assess mobility. A patient is asked to rise from a seated position in a chair, stand momentarily, walk 3 meters, turn around, walk back to the chair, turn around, and sit down. The patient is rated on a scale of 1 to 5. 1 is normal, 2 is very slightly abnormal, 3 is mildly abnormal, 4 is moderately abnormal, and 5 is severely abnormal. A patient with a score of 3 or more is at risk of falling. Normal values for various age groups have been standardized. Less than 15 seconds is a general cutoff for the upper limit of normal.

Sock Test

The Sock test is scored from 0 (normal) to 3 (worst score). The score was originally designed to evaluate the limitations caused by musculoskeletal pain. The patient simulates putting on a sock. 0: indicates the patient can perform the action with ease; 1: performs the action with effort (patients can grab their toes with their fingertips); 2: patients can reach beyond the malleoli, but cannot reach toes; 3: can hardly reach at all (able to reach malleoli only or unable to reach malleoli).

6-Minute Walk Test

This test is used to measure the response to medical interventions in moderate to severe heart/lung disease. The distance ambulated in 6 minutes is measured. Distances before and after the medical intervention can be assessed.

Suggested Readings

Crooks V, Waller S, Smith T, Hahn TJ. The use of the Karnofsky Performance Scale in determining outcomes and risk in geriatric outpatients. *J Gerontol.* 1991;46:M139–M144.

Mathias S, Nayak USL, Isaacs B. Balance in elderly patients: The "get-up and go" test. *Arch Phys Med Rehabil.* 1986;67:387–389.

Oken MM, Creech RH, Tormey DC, et al. Toxicity and response criteria of the Eastern Cooperative Oncology Group. *Am J Clin Oncol.* 1982;5:649–655.

Physical Impairments and Guidelines for Therapy Interventions and Assessments

Janet Scheetz PT

Impairments

Common impairments faced by the individual with an oncology diagnosis

Impairments exhibited are the result of the disease process itself and/or the treatment intervention such as surgery, radiation, chemotherapy, and hormonal management (see Table 5.1). Inability to perform basic and higher level functional activities can be caused by a number of impairments in cancer patients (see Table 5.2).

Table 5.1   Common Impairments Related to Type of Cancer Treatment

Common impairments	Cancer treatment modality			
	Surgery	Radiation	Chemotherapy	Hormonal
Limitation of range of motion	x	x		
Decreased muscle strength	x	x	x	
Increased soft tissue fibrosis	x	x		
Decreased aerobic capacity	x	x	x	x
Increased pain	x	x	x	x
Decreased efficiency in gait pattern to include balance and coordination	x	x	x	
Lymphedema	x	x	x	
Low vision	x	x	x	
Impaired cognition/impaired visual perceptual skills	x	x	x	x
Weight gain			x	x
Peripheral neuropathies	x		x	
Plexopathies	x	x		
Steroid myopathy			x	
Cancer-related fatigue		x	x	x
At risk for falls	x	x	x	
Osteopenia/osteoporosis	x		x	x
Osteonecrosis		x	x	
Venous thrombotic events/Pulmonary embolus	x	x	x	x
Cardiac myopathy		x	x	
Pulmonary fibrosis		x	x	
Poor motor planning	x	x	x	x

Table 5.2   Functional Deficits Related to Cancer Impairment

Functional performance deficits	Possible impairment causes
Inability to perform an efficient gait pattern	Peripheral neuropathies, poor motor planning, vision deficit, cognitive impairment, loss of strength and/or range of motion, pain in the limb or trunk, cancer-related fatigue, risk for falls, impaired divided attention
Inability to perform Basic ADL and Instrumental ADL	Cancer-related fatigue, poor motor planning, impaired working memory, weakness, poor pulmonary function, peripheral neuropathy, depression, anxiety
Inability to engage in leisure activities	Pain, impaired executive function, cardiopulmonary impairment, vision deficit, peripheral neuropathy, anxiety, depression
Inability to return to work	Cancer-related fatigue, impaired muscle endurance, distractibility, peripheral neuropathy, anxiety, depression
Inability to drive	Cognitive impairments, visual impairments, peripheral neuropathies, loss of visual perceptual skills, anxiety
Inability to return to prior roles (such as friend, cook, volunteer, mother, caregiver, etc.)	Cancer-related fatigue, cardiopulmonary impairment, peripheral neuropathy, pain, anxiety, depression

ADL, activity of daily living.

Guidelines for Therapy Interventions

Lab values

In the oncology setting it is imperative to assess the lab values of the patient prior to implementing physical therapy services. Lab values can help indicate whether therapy treatment can safely be performed (see Table 5.3).

Table 5.3   Laboratory Values and Rehabilitation Implications

Lab name	Values	MDACC values	Rehabilitation implications	Other findings
White blood cells	Normal 5,000–11,000/ mm^3	4.0–11.0 K/mcL	Risk for infections	Absolute neutrophil count of 0.5 or lower, avoid activities that increase risk of bacterial infection (swimming)
Platelets	Normal 150,000– 400,000 K/mcL	140–440 K/mcL	Less than 5 K only active assistive movements/no valsalva maneuvers Less than 20 K active movements; no resistive motions More than 50 K active resistive movements	Check for petechia Petechia is a small (1–2 mm) red or purple spot on the body, caused by a minor hemorrhage of the capillary vessel Check for any active signs of bleeding (e.g., Bleeding gums, coughing up blood, painful swollen joints, etc.)
Hemoglobin	Normal Male: 13–18 g/dL Female: 12–16 g/dL	Male: 14.0–18.0 g/dL Female: 12.0–16.0 g/dL	Less than 8 g/dL—defer therapy if symptomatic 8–10 g/dL—monitor patient closely (shortened therapy session) More than 10 g/dL—resistive exercise	Fatigue, increased rest periods, increased heart rate
Hematocrit	Normal Male: 37%–49% Female: 36%–46%	Male: 40%–54% Female: 37.0%–47.0%	Less than 20%—can result in cardiac failure/death Less than 25%—defer therapy 25%–30%—ADL and exercise, as tolerated 30%—can add resistive exercise	

Physical performance assessments (normative values as defined in the oncology population)
Objective test measures assist the physician and physical therapist in establishing, monitoring, and evaluating the progress of physical therapy interventions. Table 5.4 shows some of the test measures that have been validated in the oncology population.

Table 5.4   Functional Measures in the Oncology Setting

Test measure	Normative values	Reason for performing the test measure
6-minute walk test	1,838 feet	Assess aerobic capacity, endurance, and risk for falls
50-foot fast walk	8.43–9.32 seconds	Assess gait speed and risk for falls
Timed repeated sit to stand times two	2.19–2.73 seconds	Assess proximal strength of the lower extremities
Uni-ped stance	30 seconds	Assess balance and risk for falls
Forward reach	32.87–36.64 cm	Assess balance and risk for falls
Sock test	4.25–5.35 seconds	Assess dynamic sitting balance, visual perceptual skills, cognitive, fine motor skills, motor planning, aerobic capacity, trunk stability
Coin test (picking up 4 coins)	5.06–6.05 seconds	Cognition, vision, motor planning, fine motor, sensation

I: Background, Evaluation, and Interventions

Pulmonary Rehabilitation

Vickie R. Shannon MD

Description

Pulmonary rehabilitation (PR) is a comprehensive intervention designed to optimize functional status, reduce symptoms of chronic dyspnea and fatigue, and improve health-related quality of life (HRQoL) among patients with chronic respiratory diseases. Exercise intolerance resulting from dyspnea and fatigue may occur at any point along the cancer continuum and often persists for years after specific cancer therapies have been completed. The goals of PR are achieved through exercise training, patient self-management education, and psychosocial and behavioral interventions provided by the coordinated efforts of a multidisciplinary health care team. The multidisciplinary team typically includes physicians, nurses, physical (PT) and occupational therapists (OT), with referrals to experts in respiratory therapy (RT), exercise physiology, nutrition, psychology, and social work based on individual patient assessments and needs.

Background and Rationale for PR in Cancer: Symptom Burden in Cancer Patients

- Prevalence of fatigue: 75% (solid malignancies); 80%–90% (hematologic malignancies)
- Prevalence of dyspnea: Over 50%; Highest prevalence—lung cancer and advanced malignancies
- Chronic obstructive pulmonary disease (COPD) occurs among 80% of patients with lung cancer and compounds the symptom burden.
- Deconditioning, anxiety, and muscle weakness are common contributors to cancer-related disability.
- These symptoms adversely impact performance status, cancer treatment options, and outcomes.

Major Features of a Successful PR Program

- *Individual assessment* of needs: program should be designed to meet realistic individual goals among patients with chronic disabling disease.
- *Multidisciplinary approach*: expertise from various health care disciplines is integrated into a comprehensive, cohesive program that is tailored to the needs of each patient.

- *Attention to physical and psychosocial performance*: must address psychological as well as pathophysiologic problems that impact performance status and HRQoL.

Patient Selection Criteria

- Include any patient with chronic persistent exercise limitation despite optimal medical management.
- Referrals can be based on symptoms, not only on the magnitude of physiologic impairment.

Contraindications to PR

- Absolute
  - Severe pulmonary hypertension, refractory cor pulmonale, or exercise-induced syncope
  - Severe congestive heart failure refractory to medical management
  - Unstable coronary syndromes and/or heart disease at risk for arrhythmia or sudden death
  - Unstable skeletal disease (due to malignancy, arthritis, etc.)
- Relative
  - End-stage hepatic failure
  - Inability to learn
  - Psychiatric instability

Goals of PR in the Cancer Patient

- To restore physical activity to the highest level of independent function
- To reduce symptoms associated with activities of daily function
- To optimize HRQoL/performance status prior to and/or during cancer therapy
- To improve HRQoL/performance status following cancer therapy

Components of a Comprehensive PR Program

- Exercise training
  - General considerations in the cancer setting
    - Exercise prescriptions are based on pretreatment assessments (pulmonary function tests, 6-minute walk examination, exercise physiology testing, clinical examination).
    - Evidence-based guidelines for PR are not available in the cancer setting.

– Type of exercises
  - Stretching of accessory muscles of respiration, including chest wall
  - Endurance (aerobic) training: treadmill walking, cycle ergometry
– Benefits: increased aerobic capacity and anaerobic threshold; reduced demand and heart rate
  - Strength (resistance) training: weights, bands
– Benefits: increased muscle strength and muscle mass
  - A combination of endurance and strength training is recommended.
  - Both upper and lower extremity training are recommended.
– Exercise intensity
  - High-intensity exercise produces greater physiologic benefit.
  - A significant but lesser benefit is produced with low-intensity training, which is recommended for patients who cannot achieve high levels of exercise intensity.
– Exercise duration and frequency
  - Optimal training session duration/frequency is not established in the cancer setting. Based on the COPD literature, 60-minute sessions, given at least 3 times/week are recommended.
  - Longer programs (longer than 12 weeks) may produce more sustainable benefits than shorter ones (less than 6 weeks).
  - Interval training: promotes higher training levels in more symptomatic patients.
  - Benefits wane over time; post-PR maintenance program strategies may prolong benefits achieved in physical endurance, cognitive, psychological, and social functioning.
– Cautions
  - Safety concerns and individual patient needs/goals of PR that are unique to the cancer patient population must guide the exercise prescription and implementation of the PR program.
  - Optimal timing of PR referral relative to cancer therapy has not been established.
  - Oxygen saturation and vital signs should be monitored during exercise; telemetry monitoring should be considered for patients with a prior history of arrhythmia.
  - Sessions should be discontinued if chest pain, dizziness/lightheadedness, or palpitations develop.

  - Weight lifting or resistive exercises that require Valsalva maneuver should be avoided in patients with a history of pulmonary hypertension; low intensity exercise may be appropriate in patients with mild to moderate pulmonary hypertension.
■ Occupational therapy
  – Integrates physiological gains into functional benefits relevant to activities of daily living (ADLs).
  – Benefits achieved through functional training in ADLs, energy-conserving strategies, and the use of assistive devices.
■ Education
  – Educational topics
    - Early treatment and prevention of respiratory exacerbations
    - Breathing retraining and breathing strategies (diaphragmatic breathing, pursed-lip breathing, active expiration, paced breathing techniques, adaptive body positions)
    - Bronchial hygiene and proper use of bronchodilators
    - Nutrition
  – Educational goals
    - Better understanding of the disease process
    - Integration of disease demands into daily routines
    - Promotion of self-management skills with emphasis on illness control, self-efficacy, and adherence to therapeutic interventions
    - Knowledge of when to seek health care services
■ Psychosocial support/behavioral modification
  – Goals
    - To reduce maladaptive symptoms of anxiety, stress, and depression
    - To provide a socially supportive environment
    - To encourage stress management through relaxation training techniques
    - Tobacco cessation
  – Intervention
    - Initial assessment should include screening tools for anxiety and depression.
    - Significant other/caregiver should be interviewed to identify maladaptive behaviors at home.
    - Referrals for psychological counseling, nutrition, and social work, as indicated
    - Tobacco-cessation-program referral for active users of tobacco products

Potential Therapeutic Adjuncts to PR

- Optimization of pharmacologic therapy
  - Optimization of bronchodilator therapy in patients with airflow limitation prior to PR
  - Tiotropium bromide may improve exercisability in patients with airflow limitation.
- Supplemental oxygen
  - Recommended in patients with exercise-induced hypoxemia (SaO_2 less than 90%).
  - Gains in exercise endurance may be seen in patients who remain normoxemic during exercise, but long-term benefits and effect on other outcomes such as HRQoL have not been determined.
- Nutritional supplementation
  - No studies have evaluated weight management (gain or loss) on PR outcome.
  - Insufficient evidence to support the routine use of nutritional supplementation in PR.
- Noninvasive ventilation
  - Patients with severe lung disease may show modest gains in exercise performance.
- Anabolic agents
  - May improve muscle strength but no improvements in exercise endurance.
  - Current evidence does not support use.
  - Unsafe in patients with hormonally sensitive tumors.
- Heliox therapy
  - Combination of oxygen and helium used to decrease the work of breathing.
  - May increase exercise tolerance, but no sustained improvements in PR benefits.
- Neuromuscular stimulation (NMS)
  - May improve muscle strength/endurance, but insufficient evidence to support NMS in PR.

Clinical Outcome Assessment Tools

- Measurements of ADL and/or HRQoL
  - Chronic Respiratory Disease Questionnaire (CRQ)
  - St. George's Questionnaire
  - Borg scale

- Measurements of exercise ability
  - 6-minute walk test (6MWT)
  - Shuttle walk test
  - Cardiopulmonary exercise test

Helpful Hints

- Patients with chronic respiratory disease associated with cancer and/or its treatment may show significant physiologic and functional benefits following a program of PR.
- Current practice and expert opinion suggest that PR in these patients must be modified to include individualized PR treatment strategies specific to the disease process. This requires a careful baseline clinical examination and knowledge of the cancer type and severity, individual patient needs, functional limitation(s), and risk factors that may render PR unsafe, such as unstable bone metastases.
- Exercise training duration may be adapted to meet the patient's cancer-related needs.
  - Short duration PR (2–4 weeks) may be appropriate in cancer patients anticipating elective surgery, although the benefits of this practice have not been established in large randomized trials.
- The optimal timing of PR relative to cancer therapy has likewise not been established.

Suggested Readings

Nici L. The role of pulmonary rehabilitation in the lung cancer patient. *Semin Respir Crit Care Med.* 2009;30(6):670–674. Epub 2009 Nov 25. Review.

Quist M, Rørth M, Langer S, et al. Safety and feasibility of a combined exercise intervention for inoperable lung cancer patients undergoing chemotherapy: A pilot study. *Lung Cancer.* 2012;75(2):203–208. Epub 2011 Aug 3.

Reardon J, Casaburi R, Morgan M, et al. Pulmonary rehabilitation for COPD. *Respir Med.* 2005;99(suppl B): S19–S27. Epub 2005 Oct 25. Review.

Ries AL. Pulmonary rehabilitation: Summary of an evidence-based guideline. *Respir Care.* 2008;53(9):1203–1207. Review.

Ries AL, Bauldoff GS, Carlin BW, et al. Pulmonary rehabilitation: Joint ACCP/AACVPR evidence-based clinical practice guidelines. *Chest.* 2007;131(5 Suppl):4S–42S. Review.

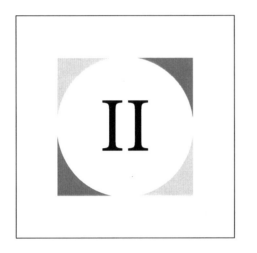

Primary Concerns
or Conditions

Bone Marrow Transplantation

Eugene Kichung Chang MD

Description

Definitive treatment for cancer involving the bone marrow (e.g., certain leukemias, lymphomas) often requires the need for bone marrow transplantation (BMT). Multifactorial issues can lead to a patient's functional decline pre and post-BMT, including secondary medical complications, toxicity from treatment, and effects from the primary cancer itself.

Types

- Allogeneic = unrelated donor
- Autologous = self as donor
- Haploidentical = "half-matched" from a sibling or parent

Epidemiology

- Each year, approximately 18,000 people in the United States are diagnosed with life-threatening illnesses that can be treated with BMT; more than 14,700 patients received bone marrow or umbilical cord transplants in 2009.
- Approximately 70% of patients do not find a matching donor within their families.

BMT Process

- Pretransplant preparative regimen (radiation and/or chemotherapy): Myeloablative versus reduced-intensity regimens to wipe out host and cancer cells prior to engrafting donor cells.
- Transplantation: Occurs through an intravenous infusion of donor stem cells, with subsequent engraftment in the host bone marrow; often requires ECOG (Eastern Cooperative Oncology Group) level of 2 or more, or able to ambulate and perform self-care independently (see Chapter 4: Performance Measures).
- Posttransplant monitoring and support: Immunosuppressive medications, regular blood work, blood transfusions ± infection prophylaxis

Medical Issues

- Graft failure or the failure of the host to accept the donor's cells, which results in a lack of normal bone marrow function
- Myelosuppression (anemia, thrombocytopenia, neutropenia)
- Immunosuppression with infection risk (EBV [Epstein-Barr virus], CMV [cytomegalovirus], viral hepatitis)
- Toxicity from treatment (mucositis, diarrhea, nausea/vomiting, peripheral neuropathy, cardiopulmonary dysfunction, steroid myopathy)
- Graft-versus-host disease (GvHD): T-cell mediated immune response in which donor graft cells recognize host cells as foreign; occurs in 20% to 50% of patients who receive stem cells from human leucocyte antigen (HLA)-identical sibling donors and in 50% to 80% of patients receiving stem cells from an HLA-mismatched sibling or an HLA-identical unrelated donor; most commonly causes skin rash, diarrhea, and/or liver dysfunction.
- Hepatic veno-occlusive disease: Occlusion of the terminal hepatic venules and hepatic sinusoids with potential for liver failure.
- Respiratory complications: pulmonary edema/hemorrhage, idiopathic pneumonia, bronchiolitis obliterans
- Infertility in up to approximately 85% of males and females post-BMT

Functional Barriers

- Asthenia
- Immobility
- Fatigue
- Poor nutrition
- Physical issues due to medical complications such as dyspnea following pneumonia
- Cognitive impairment due to radiation or chemotherapy
- Steroid myopathy: Often associated with treatment of GvHD, causing decreased proximal muscle strength, decreased mobility, strength, and endurance.
- Peripheral neuropathy: Can be due to chemotherapy, causing decreased sensation/proprioception, decreased dexterity, and foot drop.

Treatment

- Medical
  - GvHD: Treatment with high-dose corticosteroid in conjunction with steroid-sparing agent; high grade GvHD of the skin can cause nonarticular soft tissue contractures; although prevention is the key to

management, established contractures may benefit from gentle range of motion and serial casting.

– Steroid myopathy: Taper corticosteroids (if indicated), strengthening exercises, environmental adaptations (e.g., raised toilet seat, furniture)

– Peripheral neuropathy: Consider adjusting chemotherapy regimen as per primary oncologist; evaluate need for orthoses and assistive devices.

– Long term: Blood-work monitoring, reimmunization schedule, annual influenza vaccinations, mood/cognition monitoring, address issues of pain, sexual dysfunction

■ Exercises

– Avoid inactivity/immobility: Encourage aerobic conditioning exercises, strengthening and active range-of-motion throughout the pre to posttransplantation phases; be aware of platelet levels.

Consults

■ Physical medicine and rehabilitation
■ Hematology oncology (BMT/leukemia/lymphoma)
■ Radiation/medical oncology

Prognosis

■ Depends on age, cancer type, disease status at time of BMT, donor match, and severity of GvHD
■ Allogeneic BMT patients: 55% 2-year survival, 27% survival over 6 years
■ After 5 years of survival post-BMT, survival rates start to approach that of the normal population

Helpful Hints

■ Keep a high level of suspicion for potentially serious medical complications (e.g., pneumonia, sepsis) in even mildly symptomatic patients.
■ Consider fertility counseling pretransplant for sperm banking and egg cryopreservation prior to chemotherapy and/or radiation for future family planning.
■ Physiotherapy referral needed pretransplant for appropriate strengthening and conditioning exercise routines in preparation for potential functional decline given toxicity of treatment.

Suggested Reading

Gillis TA, Donovan ES. Rehabilitation following bone marrow transplantation. *Cancer.* 2001;92(4 suppl):998–1007.

Brain: Leptomeningeal Disease

Jack B. Fu MD

Description
The spread of cancer cells to the meningeal surfaces.

Etiology
- Leptomeningeal disease (LMD) arises from the spread of tumor cells into the spaces that are covered by the meninges (dura, meningeal, and pia mater).
- Tumor cells can coat the surfaces of the central nervous system.

Epidemiology
- LMD is diagnosed in 5% of patients with metastatic cancer.
- LMD may be undiagnosed in as many as 20% of patients with advanced disease.

Pathogenesis
- Arises from the hematogenous spread of tumor cells from the primary cancer site or from spreading within the central nervous system (CNS) (e.g., drop metastasis).
- Can result in disrupted cerebrospinal fluid (CSF) circulation.
- Can result in direct inflammatory effects on nerve roots and spinal nerves.
- Can result in cerebral edema.
- Direct invasion of the CNS parenchyma
- May follow surgical resection or use of chemotherapeutic agents that do not cross the blood–brain barrier.

Risk Factors
- Primary brain tumor
- Liquid tumor (lymphoma, leukemia)
- Breast cancer
- Lung cancer
- Gastrointestinal cancer

Clinical Features
- Possible meningeal signs
- New weakness/incoordination
- New or worsened bladder dysfunction
- New or worsened bowel dysfunction
- New sensory changes
- New seizures

- Neurologic symptoms may exhibit patterns that cannot be explained by one solitary lesion but by lesions throughout the nervous system.

Natural History
- A patient with known history of cancer presents with new neurologic symptoms.
- Symptom onset can be rapid or progressive.
- Sometimes patients also exhibit meningeal signs, such as headache or photophobia.
- Patients may experience neurogenic bowel and bladder.
- Gait instability, falling, and ataxia are commonly reported.

Diagnosis

Differential diagnosis
- Brain or spinal cord metastasis
- Brain abscess
- Primary brain tumor
- Brain hemorrhage
- Ischemic cerebrovascular accident
- Radiation late effects
- Chemo-brain-related cognitive changes
- Failure to thrive/malnutrition
- Steroid myopathy

History
- Known history of cancer
- Known history of recent neurologic procedure
- Progressive neurologic symptoms
- Symptoms that could be explained by multiple lesions
- Possible upper and lower motor neuron signs
- Meningeal signs, such as headache or photophobia

Examination
- Detailed neurologic examination, including sensation, cranial nerves, swallow, speech, motor exam, reflexes, and tone
- Evaluation of cognition may be indicated.

Testing
- MRI
- CT
- Lumbar puncture (LP) with CSF analysis

Pitfalls

- Many patients have clinical symptoms of LMD and have negative lumbar punctures. Clinicians often treat suspected LMD even if LP is negative.
- Prophylactic intrathecal chemotherapy is often given to liquid tumor (hematologic cancer) patients.

Treatment

Medical

- Intrathecal chemotherapy is given via an Ommaya reservoir or lumbar puncture.
- Radiation therapy can be given to treat focal areas of LMD.
- Prophylaxis against complications of immobility
- Treatment of neurogenic bowel and bladder

Surgical

- Neurosurgical evaluation is often required for placement of an Ommaya reservoir to instill intrathecal chemotherapy.

Exercises

- Exercises and therapy can address the neurologic deficits.
- Range of motion exercises for paralyzed limbs
- Training in ADLs, ambulation, transfers, and wheelchair mobility

Consults

- Physical medicine and rehabilitation
- Neurosurgery
- Neurology
- Neuropsychology
- Radiation oncology
- Oncology

Complications of treatment

- Toxicity related to the intrathecal chemotherapy can occur.
- Radiation effects can also be seen (refer to Chapter 49).

Prognosis

- Survival prognosis varies depending on primary tumor type; but in general, LMD is a poorer prognostic indicator for the patient.
- Neurologic symptoms generally improve with intrathecal chemotherapy treatment.

Helpful Hints

- These patients are at high risk for deep vein thrombosis (DVT) owing to immobility and cancer-related hypercoagulability.
- Thrombocytopenia, active bleed, or known hemorrhage on brain imaging may contraindicate pharmacologic DVT prophylaxis.
- Profound thrombocytopenia and leukopenia may significantly limit aggressive treatment of neurogenic bowel and bladder.

Suggested Readings

DeAngelis LM, Posner JB. *Neurologic Complications of Cancer.* (Contemporary neurology series) (pp. 447–510). New York, NY: Oxford University Press; 2009.

Glass JP, Melamed MF, Chernik NL, et al. Malignant cells in cerebrospinal fluid (CSF): The meaning of a positive CSF cytology. *Neurology.* 1979;29(10):1369–1375.

Groves MD. Leptomeningeal disease. *Neurosurg Clin N Am.* 2011;22(1):67–78, vii. doi: 10.1016/j.nec.2010.08.006

II: Primary Concerns or Conditions

Brain: Metastatic Tumors

Jack B. Fu MD

Description
Metastatic brain tumors originate from other cancers.

Etiology
- Tumors' cells infiltrate the blood–brain barrier, typically by hematogenous spread.
- The metastatic lesion can directly invade surrounding brain tissue.
- Pressure on surrounding brain tissue can result in neurologic symptoms.
- Pressure on surrounding brain tissue can result in mass effect and hydrocephalus.

Epidemiology
- Much more common than primary brain tumors (20%–50% of autopsied cancer patients have brain metastases).
- More than half of people with metastatic brain tumors have multiple lesions (tumors).
- 100,000 to 150,000 metastatic brain tumors are diagnosed each year in the United States.

Pathogenesis
- These tumors arise from the hematogenous spread of tumor cells from the primary cancer site.
- Because many chemotherapy agents do not cross the blood–brain barrier, they often escape treatment.

Risk Factors
- Lung cancer
- Breast cancer
- Colon cancer
- Renal cancer
- Melanoma

Clinical Features
- Neurologic symptoms are often gradual in onset, usually over weeks to months in a patient with a known cancer history.
- However, sudden onset of neurologic symptoms such as seizures and visual loss is reported.
- Patients may exhibit upper motor neuron signs.
- Headache, visual loss, confusion, seizures, and incoordination are also commonly reported.
- Patients often have more than one metastatic brain lesion at the time of diagnosis.

Natural History
- Typically, symptoms gradually progress until the patient seeks medical attention.
- In some patients, the metastatic brain lesion is the first sign of cancer that is diagnosed.

Diagnosis
Differential diagnosis
- Seizure
- Brain abscess
- Primary brain tumor
- Brain hemorrhage
- Ischemic cerebrovascular accident
- Radiation late effects
- Chemo-brain-related cognitive changes

History
- Patients with a known diagnosis of cancer
- Headaches
- Seizures
- Weakness
- Incoordination
- Visual changes

Examination
- Detailed neurologic examination, including sensation and cranial nerves, swallow, speech, motor exam, reflexes, and tone
- Evaluation of cognition may be indicated.

Testing
- MRI
- CT

Pitfalls
- Biopsy is not always warranted but can help in confirming the diagnosis.

Treatment
Medical
- Treatment is dependent on tumor type.
- Radiation therapy may be indicated. Whole-brain radiation is used for widespread or multiple lesions. Stereotactic radiosurgery may be used for small isolated lesions or lesions that are difficult to resect surgically.
- Systemic chemotherapy may also be needed in many cases.

Surgical

- Neurosurgical resection may be performed if the location is amenable to resection and it is causing significant symptoms.
- Surgery may be deferred if the lesions are too widespread, difficult to resect, or too small.

Exercises

- Exercises and therapy should address the neurologic deficits.
- Range of motion exercises for paralyzed limbs
- Training in activities of daily living, ambulation, transfers, and wheelchair mobility

Consults

- Physical medicine and rehabilitation
- Neurosurgery
- Neurology
- Neuropsychology
- Radiation oncology
- Oncology

Complications of treatment

- Surgical resection can result in worsening or new neurologic symptoms. However, patients often experience improvement as swelling and edema subside.
- Radiation therapy often causes fatigue immediately after treatment. Many patients also suffer headache exacerbations.

Prognosis

- Survival prognosis varies depending on the primary tumor type; but in general, metastases are a poorer prognostic indicator for the patient. Often, tumors will recur at the metastatic site.
- Neurologic prognosis is dependent on the response of the lesions to radiation treatment or success of surgical resection.

Helpful Hints

- These patients are at high risk for deep vein thrombosis (DVT) due to immobility and cancer-related hypercoagulability.
- Thrombocytopenia, active bleed, or known hemorrhage on brain imaging may contraindicate pharmacologic DVT prophylaxis.
- Profound thrombocytopenia and leukopenia may significantly limit aggressive treatment of neurogenic bowel and bladder.

Suggested Readings

Wen P, Schiff D, Kesari S, et al. Medical management of patients with brain tumors. *J Neurooncol.* 2006;80:313–332.

Yung WK, Kunschner LJ, et al. Intracranial metastases. In: Levin VA, ed. *Cancer in the Nervous System.* New York, NY: Oxford University Press; 2002:321–340.

II: Primary Concerns or Conditions

Brain: Primary Tumors

Jack B. Fu MD

Description
Primary brain tumors arise from within the brain.

Etiology/Types
- Over 120 different types of primary brain tumors exist.
- Tumors are divided into World Health Organization (WHO) grades.
- Many also occur in the spinal cord.
- The most commonly encountered brain tumor in adults is high-grade astrocytomas.
- Others include oligodendroglioma, meningioma, craniopharyngioma, pituitary tumors, ependymoma, schwannoma, and central nervous system lymphoma.
- Childhood primary brain tumors include medulloblastoma, brain stem glioma, low-grade astrocytoma, craniopharyngioma, ependymoma, and pineal tumor.
- Low-grade WHO astrocytomas are: grade I (pilocytic, subependymal, and pleomorphic xanthoastrocytoma) and grade II (protoplasmic, gemistocytic, fibrillary, diffuse, and mixed).
- High-grade WHO astrocytomas are: grade III (anaplastic) and grade IV (glioblastoma multiforme [GBM]).
- The grade is based on pathologic findings. Generally, high-grade astrocytomas have a greater degree of pleomorphism, hyperchromatism, and mitosis.

Epidemiology
- Primary brain tumor incidence is estimated to be 130.8 per 100,000 individuals.
- High-grade astrocytomas account for 80% of all brain tumors in adults and have an incidence rate in the United States of 2 to 3 per 100,000 compared with 0.6 per 100,000 for low-grade astrocytomas.
- Low-grade astrocytomas are more common in younger patients (often in childhood) and high-grade astrocytomas are more common in older patients (highest incidence in adults of 50–59 years old).

Pathogenesis
- Arise from cells in the brain
- Can arise from meninges, brain, and glands

Risk Factors
- Primary radiation for cancer treatment
- Occupational radiation exposure
- Genetic predisposition including:
  - Neurofibromatosis
  - von-Hippel Lindau
  - Turcot
  - Li-Fraumeni
- Some families have higher risk, but this is uncommon.

Clinical Features
Neurologic symptoms often progress gradually, usually over weeks to months. However, a sudden onset of neurologic symptoms, such as seizures and visual loss, is reported.

- Patients may exhibit upper motor neuron signs.
- Headache
- Visual loss
- Confusion
- Seizures
- Weakness
- Incoordination

Natural History
- Symptoms gradually progress until patients seek medical attention.
- Often times, tumors are initially mistaken for the more common cerebrovascular accident, owing to their often similar neurologic findings.

Diagnosis

Differential diagnosis
- Cerebrovascular accident
- Brain abscess
- Metastatic brain lesion
- Seizure

History
- Headaches
- Seizures
- Weakness
- Incoordination
- Visual changes
- Cognitive changes

Examination

- Detailed neurologic examination, including sensation and cranial nerves, swallow, speech, motor exam, reflexes, and tone
- Evaluation of cognition may be indicated.

Testing

- MRI
- CT

Pitfalls

- Pathology biopsy results are needed before chemotherapy and radiation initiation.
- Mistaking a primary tumor for a stroke

Treatment

Medical/Surgical/Radiation/Chemotherapy

- Treatment is dependent on tumor type.
- Surgical resection is generally the initial treatment for brain tumors, followed by medical treatment.
- If the tumor is unresectable or difficult to resect, radiation therapy may be the initial treatment.
- Effort is made to remove as much tumor as is safely possible while minimizing neurologic effects.
- Repeat surgical resections are not uncommon for these patients if and when a tumor recurs.
- At times, ventriculoperitoneal shunts may be necessary for hydrocephalus.
- Surgical resection can result in worsening or new neurologic symptoms. However, patients often experience improvement as swelling and edema subside.
- Radiation therapy often causes fatigue immediately after treatment. Many patients also suffer headache exacerbations.

- For high-grade astrocytomas, current standard of care is surgical resection followed by radiation and temozolamide.
  - Oral temozolamide chemotherapy often results in nausea, vomiting, poor appetite, weight loss, and fatigue. Active therapy participation may be difficult when patients are taking the medication.

Exercises

- Exercises and therapy should address the neurologic deficits.
- Range of motion exercises for paralyzed limbs
- Training in activities of daily living, ambulation, transfers, and wheelchair mobility

Consults

- Physical medicine and rehabilitation
- Neurosurgery
- Neurooncology
- Neuropsychology
- Radiation oncology

Prognosis

- Prognosis varies depending on tumor type.
- Median lifespan for grade IV GBM, the most common adult tumor, is 12 to 15 months from the time of diagnosis or treatment.

Helpful Hint

- Pharmacologic deep venous thrombosis prophylaxis is neurosurgeon dependent. These patients are at high risk for venous thromboembolic disease.

Suggested Readings

Berger MS, Leibel SA, Bruner JM, et al. Primary cerebral tumors. In: Levin VA, ed. *Cancer in the Nervous System* (pp. 88–90). New York, NY: Oxford University Press; 2002.

Wen P, Schiff D, Kesari S, et al. Medical management of patients with brain tumors. *J Neurooncol.* 2006;80:313–332.

II: Primary Concerns or Conditions

Hematologic Cancer

Benedict Konzen MD

Description

For treatment purposes, cancer patients are referred to as having either a solid or liquid tumor. Liquid tumors refer to tumors of the blood, bone marrow, and lymph nodes. These liquid (or hematologic) tumors include:

- Myelodysplastic disorders: trilineage cellular dyscrasias
- Leukemias: acute or chronic in nature and involving the leukocytes
- Myeloma: a plasma cell dyscrasia
- Lymphoma (referred to as non-Hodgkin vs. Hodgkin); lymphomas arise from the T- or B-lymphocyte.

Epidemiology

- 61,000 people are diagnosed with blood cancers each year in the United States.
- The etiology of liquid tumors is not entirely clear. There have been links to chronic benzene exposure (e.g., in cigarette smoke) and from exposures to large doses of radiation.

Pathogenesis

- Nonrandom chromosome changes have been identified in a number of malignant human tumors.
  - Chronic myeloid leukemia has a consistent translocation t(9;22) (q34;q11), which occurs in 93% of all Ph1 positive patients.
  - In B-cell acute lymphoblastic leukemia, there is consistent change involving 8q24.
  - The challenge for the future will be to define the genes located at the sites of consistent translocations.

Clinical Features

- A patient's symptoms may be nonspecific: fatigue, weight loss, limited endurance, night sweats, bruising, abdominal fullness (hepato-splenomegaly), bone pain, fracture, irritability and/or confusion, nonhealing wounds, recurrent infections, or epistaxis.
- Blood work may demonstrate a leukocytosis or anemia.
- Imaging studies may demonstrate lytic lesions of the bone; or diffuse involvement of the central nervous system (leptomeningeal disease).

Diagnosis

- Workup will often entail extensive blood work; peripheral smears, bone marrow biopsy, and aspirate; radiographic imaging/staging; evaluation for stem cell transplantation and ancillary consultation with specialists in allied fields of internal medicine, infectious diseases, cardiology, endocrinology, cardiopulmonary medicine, and physical medicine.

Treatment

- Treatment is often based on the hematologic disorder.
- Treatment may involve established chemotherapy, chemoradiation regimens, or new protocol/targeted treatments.
- Ultimately, a patient may require either an autologous (from one's self) or an allogeneic (from an HLA-identically matched) donor stem cell transplant.

Side effects of treatment

- Anemia
- Bleeding from thrombocytopenia
- Poor wound and skin healing
- Infection
- Immunosuppression
- Graft-versus-host disease in stem cell transplant patients
- Alterations in memory, concentration, and insight
- Stroke
- Chemotherapy- or radiation-induced radiculopathy or neuropathy
- Malnutrition
- Dehydration
- Organ system failure (e.g., cardiomyopathy or renal insufficiency)
- Platelet or transfusion dependency

Implications for Rehabilitation

- Rehabilitation requires intensive involvement with physical and occupational therapists, psychologists, speech pathologists, and nutritionists.
- Physiatrists must be aware of numerous physiologic parameters, such as pancytopenia, and electrolyte disturbances, such as hypercalcemia or hypomagnesemia.
- Physiatrist must be aware of chemotherapy-induced toxicity, which may affect cardiac, renal, neurologic, and/or cognitive functioning.

Rehabilitation concerns

- The hematologic patient often is immunosuppressed, fatigued, and may have persistent pain, depression, anxiety, anhedonia, insomnia, dyspnea, and anorexia/cachexia.
- These patients often have recurrent fever, infection, anemia, constipation, and/or diarrhea, malnutrition, and dehydration.
- Pain may be musculoskeletal or neuropathic in origin. Sustained and immediate release opioid preparations (morphine, hydromorphone, methadone) and neuropathic agents (pregabalin, gabapentin, duloxetine) often are used in combination to avoid undertreating pain.
- Patients who are in pain will be less receptive to mobilization from either their bed or a sedentary position. Immobility will lead to potential contractures, impingements, wounds (decubiti), poor hygiene, and infections/pneumonia.
- In cases of stem-cell transplant patients, graft-versus-host disease may alter the architecture of the skin and joints. Without range of motion, these patients may face the sequelae of contractures and impingement syndromes.
- Constipation is often overlooked. A thorough understanding of a patient's bowel routine and proactive initiation of a bowel program can greatly reduce patient suffering and constipation-related costs.
- Anemic, malnourished, and dehydrated patients will be fatigued. Maximizing these parameters along with improving access to therapy services will help alleviate perceived/observed fatigue.

- The liquid tumor patient is prone to infection with both nosocomial and rare pathogens. Especially at risk is the allogeneic stem cell patient, who has a fledgling immune system.

Helpful Hints

- Hematologic patients require proactive medical care. In general, most cancer patients need to maintain a healthy lifestyle, including smoking cessation, decreasing alcohol consumption, maintaining a good diet, incorporating adequate rest and exercise, and attempting to ameliorate life's stressors.
- Anemia may also be due to a nutritional deficiency, bleeding from a gastrointestinal source, or anticoagulation therapy.

Suggested Readings

Adamsen L, Midtgaard J, Rorth M, et al. Feasibility, physical capacity and health benefits of a multidimensional exercise program for cancer patients undergoing chemotherapy. *Support Care Cancer.* 2003 Nov;11(11):707–716.

Jarden M, Adamsen L, Kjeldsen L. The emerging role of exercise and health counseling in patients with acute leukemia undergoing chemotherapy during outpatient management. *Leuk Res.* 2013 Feb;37(2):155–161.

NCCN.com, National Comprehensive Cancer Network. *The Difference Between Liquid and Solid Tumors.* Retrieved from http://nccn.com/component/content/article/54-cancer-basics/1042-liquid-versus-solid-tumors.html. Accessed February 26, 2013.

Rowley JD. Chromosome abnormalities in leukemia and lymphoma. *Ann Clin Lab Sci.* 1983 Mar–Apr; 13(2):87–94.

Metastatic Bone Disease: Physiatric Perspective

Rajesh R. Yadav MD

Description

- Metastatic bone disease in cancer patients can lead to significant pain, hypercalcemia, pathologic fractures, spinal cord compression, and functional limitations.

Epidemiology

- Of over 1.2 million patients diagnosed with cancer annually in the United States, approximately 600,000 have tumors with predilection for metastasis to the bone.
- Skeletal involvement occurs in 30% to 70% of all cancer patients.
- Commonly occurs in the common cancers: in 65% to 75% of prostate and breast cancer patients and in 30% to 40% of lung cancer patients.

Clinical Features

- Pain with palpation along affected area
- Decreased range of motion about affected joints
- Decreased ability to bear weight
- Decreased strength, especially with fear of exacerbating pain
- Decreased functional status, including ability to lie down, sit, and ambulate

Pathogenesis

- Metastatic cells intrude the bone marrow cavity where they form a secondary lesion.
- Spread may occur via Batson's vertebral venous plexus, lymphatic, and hematogenous routes.
- The dynamic process of bone resorption and formation is affected in cancer.
- The lesions can be classified as osteolytic, osteosclerotic, or mixed lesions.
- Osseous metastases often occur along the axial skeleton, including the skull, spine, and at proximal joints, such as the hips and shoulders.
- Breast cancers typically produce osteolytic activity owing to stimulation of osteoclasts, the bone-resorbing cells, and appear as radiolucent areas.
- Osteolytic areas may fracture even in the absence of trauma.
- Osteosclerotic metastases are associated with prostate cancer. They occur owing to stimulation of osteoblasts and thus lead to increased bone formation.
- Osteosclerotic lesions have poorly organized microstructure, increasing the risk of pathologic fractures.
- Spinal cord compression may occur owing to spinal instability.

Risk Factors

- Osseous metastases risk varies based on the tumor type:
  - Breast—73%
  - Prostate—68%
  - Thyroid—42%
  - Kidney—35%
  - Lung—36%
  - Gastrointestinal tract—5%

Diagnosis

Differential diagnosis

- Initial workup with plain radiographs may not reveal a metastatic lesion and can be confused with local musculoskeletal injury.
- Neuropathic pain with nerve, root, or plexus injury can also produce pain owing to neoplastic infiltration of these structures.

History

- Although many metastatic bone lesions cause no or few symptoms, pain is often the most common symptom.
- Most common cause of chronic pain in cancer patients.
- Pain may vary from intermittent and indolent to sharp, severe, and radiating.
- Pain may be worse at night in a recumbent position.
- Alteration in gait with lower body involvement due to metastatic lesion is not unusual.
- Neurologic symptoms can occur with vertebral metastases, which can lead to spinal instability or spinal cord compression.

Examination

- If pain is present, then decreased range of motion and strength may be seen.
- Patient may have pain with weight bearing and manual muscle testing.

- Focal pain with palpation along the bone
- Decreased strength and sensation with neurologic involvement, including spinal cord injury
- There are various criteria for determining fracture risk, and orthopedic consultation is helpful.

Testing
- Plain radiographs may reveal the tumor but up to 50% of bone mass may be lost before changes may be appreciated.
- Radiographic exam, including CT scans, reveals presence of metastatic bony disease.
- A technetium bone can be used to screen for additional bony lesions and measure bone remodeling. This test also can help indicate the response of the surrounding bone to the lesion. The results are sensitive but not specific for tumors. Multiple areas of uptake may suggest metastatic disease.
- Skeletal survey can be helpful with osteoblastic lesions and is often used with multiple myeloma and breast cancer patients.
- Serum protein electrophoresis can be helpful with diagnosis of multiple myeloma.
- CT scan and MRI can further characterize the lesion not well seen on plain radiograph.
- CT scan is useful in evaluating integrating of bony cortex and is more useful than MRI in assessment of lesions at risk for fracture.
- MRI scan with gadolinium is sensitive for detection of metastatic disease and for evaluation of intramedullary and extramedullary extent, the degree of cortical, periosteal, and extent of soft tissue involvement. It is most useful in assessment of spinal metastases and surrounding tissues.
- Bone biopsy can be used sometimes to confirm diagnosis of metastatic disease prior to more definitive treatment. Indications include appearance of possible metastatic lesions, suspicious lesions without cancer, and patients with a history of more than one primary tumor.

Treatment

Medical
- Multidisciplinary approach to treatment.
- Goals include improvement in general health, control of local symptoms, and treatment of underlying disease.
- Nutrition:
  - With advanced cancer and osseous metastases, malnutrition may be a concern. Patients may have lost significant weight. The malnutrition further

compromises decreased strength, fatigue, function, and any postoperative healing.
- Psychosocial aspects of disease:
  - Depression and anxiety are seen frequently with advanced disease, altered function, pain, and hospitalizations. Inability to interact socially in a more normal manner, work fully, financial pressures, drive, or enjoy leisurely activities impair well-being of the patients as well.
- Bone marrow suppression
- Electrolyte and mineral balance may be abnormal in patients with widespread disease.
- Avoidance of complications such as pressure ulcers and deep venous thrombosis are major concerns.
- Nonoperative treatment includes:
  - Radiation—can provide effective pain relief and functional improvement for up to 1 year in 80% of patients with radiosensitive tumors.
  - Thermal ablation may be an alternative to irradiation and surgery for metastatic lesions to the spine, pelvis, and long bones.
  - Chemotherapy
  - Chemoablation:
    - Refers to injection of tissue-lethal solution into the targeted lesion to achieve in situ tissue necrosis. Some of these agents include ethanol, hypertonic saline, and acetic acid solution.
  - Radiofrequency ablation:
    - This process refers to destruction of a small tumor by using heat generated from high frequency alternating current and is most often used with lung, liver, kidney, and bone tumors.
  - Endocrine therapy:
    - In women, use of antiestrogen tamoxifen and specific aromatase inhibitors for appropriate patients.
    - In men, orchiectomy, use of luteinizing hormone releasing hormone analogs (leuprolide) and antiandrogens may be appropriate.
  - Supportive care measures:
    - Analgesics, including opiates, nonsteroidal anti-inflammation drugs (NSAIDs), corticosteroids, anticonvulsants
    - Nonpharmacologic management of pain—nerve blocks, surgery, neurostimulatory, and physiatric techniques
    - Bisphosphonates—inhibition of tumor osteolysis: pamidronate and zoledronic acid
    - Acupuncture

– Rehabilitation:
  - Restrictions with range of motion and weight bearing are often instituted if there is weight bearing pain or risk for fracture based on imaging.
  - Use of an orthotic device may be helpful in limiting range of motion in the spine or joint.
    ○ The spinal orthotic should extend at least a few segments above and below the lesion(s).
  - Decreased weight bearing with the use of adaptive equipment such as a walker can improve pain.
  - Teaching appropriate rehabilitation techniques and training family members improves functional outcome.

Surgery

- Factors to be considered are tumor location, extent of bone destruction, general condition of the patient, prior irradiation, and expected survival. Surgical criteria may include:
  – Pain with weight bearing
  – Neurological compromise
  – Impending fracture:
    - Various criteria, including size of the lesions on imaging studies, and these may include:
      ○ more than 2 to 3 cm in lower extremity
      ○ 3.0 cm or more in upper extremity
      ○ more than 50% bony cortex involvement
      ○ more than 50% to 60% cross-sectional diameter—intramedullary lesion
- Indications include intractable pain unresponsive to nonoperative measures, existence of actively growing tumor resistant to other treatments, spinal instability, and neural compromise.
- Tumor resection, joint replacement, and hardware placement and the use of methylmethacrylate are common.
  – With metastatic spinal surgery for decompression, reconstruction may involve use of expandable titanium cages especially after vertebrectomy. These porous titanium cylinders that are placed can be filled with bone graft, which can grow through the openings. Screw and rod construct may be needed for extra support. These patients may not need postoperative back bracing.
  – Patients with pathologic fractures may benefit from surgical stabilization for pain control and better quality of life. Often, these fractures are managed with intramedullary nail, but if a fracture is not amenable to intramedullary nailing, a long spanning plate may be used.
- Preoperative arterial embolization is a valuable tool for highly vascular metastatic tumors, such as renal cell carcinoma.
- Percutaneous vertebroplasty and kyphoplasty
  – 75% of patients reported relief at 6 months

Prognosis

- The median survival time from diagnosis of bony lesions varies by tumor type.
- With prostate or breast cancer survival may be measurable in years.
- In contrast, with advanced lung cancer, median survival time is in months.
- Prognosis is often worse with the presence of extraosseous and osseous metastases compared to osseous metastases alone.

Helpful Hints

- Early diagnosis and treatment minimizes morbidity and improves functional outcomes.
- Decreased weight bearing with assistive devices can help prolong function with painful lesions.

Suggested Readings

Clezardin P, Teti A. Bone metastasis: Pathogenesis and therapeutic implications. *Clin Exp Metastasis.* 2007;24:599–608.

Coleman RE. Clinical features of metastatic bone disease and risk of skeletal morbidity. *Clin Cancer Res.* 2006;12:6243S–6249S.

Papagelopoulos PJ, Savvidou OD, Galanis EC, et al. Advances and challenges in diagnosis and management of skeletal metastases. *Orthopedics.* 2006;29:609–620.

Yu HM, Tsai Y, Hoffe SE. Overview of diagnosis and management of metastatic disease to bone. *Cancer Control.* 2012;19:84–91.

Metastatic Bone Disease: Surgical Perspective

Annie Arteau MD ■ Valerae O. Lewis MD

Epidemiology

- Over 1.5 million new cases of cancer are diagnosed each year in the United States.
- 50% metastasize to the bone.
  - 50% of these metastasize to the lower extremity and pelvis.
  - 20% metastasize to the upper extremity.
- 25% of carcinomas present with osseous lesions.
- 10% to 15% of metastases of unknown primary origin are osseous.
- Most common metastases to bone are breast, prostate, lung, thyroid, and renal carcinoma.

Solitary bone lesion

- Cannot assume lesion is metastatic even in the context of documented malignancy.
- Single metastasis is rare, however.
  - After the age of 40, metastatic lesion to bone is 500 times more frequent than primary bone sarcoma.
  - A second malignancy or a bone sarcoma is in the differential.
    - Treatments differ significantly.
- Biopsy to obtain firm diagnosis *before* definitive treatment, including surgery.
- Infection, myeloma, lymphoma, and metabolic bone diseases are always in the differential.

Pathogenesis

- Tumor cell production of IL-6, IL-11, PTHrP, and other mediators is responsible for osteoclast activation, differentiation, and bone resorption.

Diagnosis

- In the context of skeletal metastasis of unknown origin, a complete history, physical exam, laboratory studies, chest-abdomen-pelvis CT scan, bone scan, and biopsy can identify the primary site in 85% of the cases.

History

- Pain
  - Night pain is characteristic of pathological process.
  - Typically difficult to relieve with conventional pain medicine.

- Functional appendicular pain is related to decrease in cortical structural integrity.
- Extremity
  - Painful joint range of motion
  - New mass
  - Decreased strength
  - Limp/antalgic gait
- Spinal lesion with epidural extension
  - Progressive weaknesses
  - Loss of sphincter control
  - Gait disturbances
- Constitutional symptoms: weight loss, night sweats, and general fatigue are usually documented.
- Meticulous review of all systems

Examination

- Observation
  - Gait
  - Skin changes or redness
  - Deformity or mass
  - Muscle atrophy
- Palpation
  - Tenderness
  - Muscle spasm
- Range-of-motion assessment
  - Active and passive range of motion
- Complete neurologic evaluation
  - Motor exam—differentiate weakness versus pain
  - Sensation
  - Reflexes
    - Including perineum and sphincter exam
  - Vascular exam

Objectives

- Find a primary carcinoma.
- Rule out a nonsolid tumor origin for bone lesion (leukemia, multiple myeloma).
- Rule out a bone infection.
- Assess malignancy systemic effect on marrow function, electrolyte balance, and nutritional status.

Laboratory testing

- Complete blood count—marrow aplasia can result in abnormal white count and abnormal lymphocytic population.
- Erythrocyte sedimentation rate (ESR) and C-reactive protein (CRP)—can be elevated in infectious process and inflammatory or reactive process.
- Serum and urinary protein electrophoresis—can be abnormal in multiple myeloma.
- Liver enzymes and alkaline phosphatase—can be abnormal in digestive neoplasia as well as with other digestive pathology.
- Prostate-specific antigen (PSA)—prostate origin of bone metastasis is frequent.
- Thyroid-stimulating hormone (TSH), T4, and T3—abnormalities can lead to further workup for thyroid malignancy.
- Basic biochemistry, including serum calcium, magnesium, and phosphorus—assess primary hyperparathyroidism, sodium imbalance, and hypercalcemia related to malignancy
  - Malignancy-related hypercalcemia can be fatal.
- Albumin, prealbumin levels, and protein count—assess nutritional status.

Imaging studies

- Radiographs—gold standard
  - x-ray with two orthogonal views of the entire affected bone:
    - Visualize joint above and below the lesion.
    - Multiple metastases can occur in the same bone.
  - Fast
  - Inexpensive
  - Readily available
  - Determination of fracture risk
- CT scan
  - Cortical integrity assessment
  - Subtle bone destruction
  - Bone mineralization
  - Bone destruction in complex anatomic locations like pelvis, shoulder girdle, or spine
- MRI
  - Evaluate bone marrow/integrity.
  - Evaluate extent and location of soft tissue mass.
    - Soft tissue extension and relationship to neurovascular structures
  - Distinguish fractures due to osteoporosis from those due to tumors
  - Assess epidural extension.
- Bone scan
  - Sensitive but nonspecific

  - Assesses metabolic function of the lesion not structural integrity of the bone:
    - Synchronous lesions may be clinically silent.
    - Complementary x-rays should be ordered based on bone scan findings.
- Skeletal survey
  - Assess for metastatic lesions with cold bone scan.
  - Useful for lesions in which osteoclastic activity is dominant:
    - Multiple myeloma
    - Renal cell carcinoma
    - Lung carcinoma
- Chest, abdomen, and pelvis CT scan
  - In the context of solitary bone lesion:
    - Evaluate for primary disease.
    - Assess metastatic spread.
  - In the context of well-documented malignancy:
    - To assess metastatic spread/restage

Treatment

Systemic therapy for bone metastases

- Cytotoxic chemotherapy optimization
- Endocrine therapy for sensitive tumors
- Bisphosphonates
  - Bind to bone and promote osteoclast apoptotic death
  - Antitumor effect
  - Significantly lowers bone-related events in metastatic disease.

Impending fracture

- Fracture that will likely occur with physiologic loading
- Bone lesions should be addressed.
  - Weight-bearing bones should be surgically treated if life expectancy is over 1 month.
  - Nonweight-bearing bones should be surgically treated if life expectancy is over 3 months.

Benefits of prophylactic fixation of impending fractures

- Decreased perioperative morbidity/pain
- Virginal operative field
- More thorough procedure
- Control
- Shorter operating room time
- Faster recovery
- Shorter hospitalization
- Decreased narcotic utilization
- Can coordinate with medical treatment

Harington's criteria for prophylactic surgery

- More than 50% bone diameter cortical destruction
- More than 2.5-cm lesion or 50% to 75% metaphyseal bone destruction

- Persistent pain after radiation therapy
- Life expectancy of more than 1 to 2 months

Patient selection for nonoperative versus operative treatment of pathological fracture

Nonoperative
- Nondisplaced
- Nonweight-bearing bone
- Medically ill
- Short life expectancy

Operative
- Displaced
- Weight-bearing bone
- Medically well
- Longer life expectancy

Nonoperative treatment options
- Activity modification
- Pain medication
- Immobilization/functional bracing
- Minimally invasive techniques
  - Radiofrequency ablation, cryotherapy
- Radiation therapy

Nonoperative complications
- Atrophy and weakness
- Atelectasis
- Thromboembolic disease

Surgical intervention needed
- Impending pathological fracture
- Significant symptomatic joint destruction
- Pathologic fracture of lower extremity if life expectancy is greater than 1 month
- Pathologic fracture of upper extremity if life expectancy is greater than 3 months
  - Considerations: Fracture type, significant functional compromise, need of assistive device for ambulation and expected response to conservative treatment
- Progressive myelopathy with more than 3 to 6 months of life expectancy
- Failure of nonsurgical treatment

Goals of surgical treatment
- Alleviate pain
- Restore skeletal stability
- Regain function or ambulation

Surgical options
- Depend on location, tissue histology, remaining bone stock

- Diaphyseal lesions
  - Prophylactic or therapeutic nailing/rodding
  - Adjunctive curettage and cementation
    - Provides immediate mechanical strength
    - Decreases the local tumor volume
    - Useful for radio-insensitive tumors like renal cell carcinoma or large defects
- Epiphyseal or metaphyseal lesions
  - Curettage and cementation ± plate fixation
  - Resection and endoprosthetic reconstruction
- Acetabular lesions
  - Curettage and cementation and rebar fixation
  - Resection arthroplasty
  - Complex cementation and endoprosthetic reconstruction
- Radical resection of metastasis does not affect the prognosis.
  - Renal cell carcinoma may be an exception
- Percutaneous noninvasive procedures (cementoplasty, cryoplasty, and radiofrequency ablation)
  - Focal spinal lesions
  - Nonweight-bearing areas (metaphysis, flat bones, acetabulum)
- Spinal lesion
  - Decompression with or without spinal stabilization for epidural metastatic extension with myelopathy unresponsive to medical treatment
  - Instrumentation for structurally compromised spine

Rehabilitation
- Goal: optimization of pain-free range of motion, ambulation, and quality of life
- Comprehensive rehabilitation program is based on the anatomic location, reconstruction operation performed, remaining bone stock, and overall patient health status.
- Immediate postoperative rehabilitation: breathing, isometric exercises, chair mobilization
- Upper extremity:
  - Wrist and elbow range of motion, swelling control
  - Progressive shoulder range of motion as tolerated, isometric exercises and progressive gentle strengthening if fixation done
    - If endoprosthetic reconstruction performed shoulder is immobilized.
      - Abduction brace worn for about 6 weeks
      - Keeps shoulder girdle muscles at shortest length (contraction length)
      - Allow scar tissue to form and provide stability to the prosthesis.

- Lower extremity
  - Strengthening
    - Isometric quadriceps and hip flexor strengthening.
  - Mobilization
    - Weight bearing is dependent on reconstruction performed
    - Fall prevention
    - Prevent Achilles tendon contracture and pressure sores.
  - Assistive devices
    - Discontinue when muscle control, equilibrium, and strength are regained.
      o Some patients need lifelong assistive device.
  - Hip abduction brace or knee immobilizer is often prescribed for about 6 weeks to allow surgical site healing and to prevent instability.

Prognosis

Metastatic bone involvement can significantly impact survival (see Table 13.1).

Table 13.1   Effect of Presenting Bone Metastases on Survival

Overall 5-year carcinoma survival rate (%)	
Prostate	93
Breast	85
Lung	14
Renal	61
Thyroid	95

Overall 5-year survival rate with presenting bone metastases (%)	
Prostate	33
Breast	22
Lung	2
Renal	10
Thyroid	44

- Healed lesions after prophylactic or therapeutic nailing should achieve pain-free ambulation and range of motion.
- Endoprosthetic reconstruction of the proximal femur or proximal humerus achieves pain relief but expected function is relatively poor and related to bone and muscles resection (rotator cuff, hip abductors). Instability is a concern after proximal femur resection and reconstruction.
- Spinal cord recovery is unpredictable after spinal decompression.

Helpful Hints

- Underestimation of patient survival may lead to suboptimal local treatment.
- Tragic mistake to spare operation when the procedure can make an important improvement in the quality of the patient's remaining life.

Suggested Readings

Biermann JS, Holt GE, Lewis VO, et al. Metastatic bone disease: Diagnosis, evaluation, and treatment. *J Bone Joint Surg Am.* 2009;91(6):1518–1530.

Body JJ, Mancini I. Bisphosphonates for cancer patients: Why, how, and when? *Support Care Cancer.* 2002;10(5): 399–407.

Callaway GH, Healey JH. Surgical management of metastatic carcinoma. *Curr Opin Orthop.* 1990;1:416–422.

Hong J, Cabe GD, Tedrow JR, et al. Failure of trabecular bone with simulated lytic defects can be predicted non-invasively by structural analysis. *J Orthop Res.* 2004;22:479–486.

Mirels H. Metastatic disease in long bones: A proposed scoring system for diagnosing impending pathologic fractures. *Clin Orthop Relat Res.* 2003;(415 suppl):S4–S13.

Rougraff BT, Kneisl JS, Simon MA. Skeletal metastases of unknown origin. A prospective study of a diagnostic strategy. *J Bone Joint Surg Am.* 1993;75:1276–1281.

Neurofibromatosis Type 1 and Type 2

An Ngo DO

Description
- Neurofibromatosis type 1 (NF1) and neurofibromatosis type 2 (NF2) are autosomal dominant disorders marked by neurogenic tumors arising from the neural sheath cells of peripheral and cranial nerves, producing skin and bone deformities.
- These patients can have significant rehabilitation needs that are often overlooked.

Etiology/Types
- NF1: Mutation of the NF1 gene on chromosome 17q11.2, which encodes for the protein neurofibromin.
- NF2: Mutation of the NF2 gene on chromosome 22q12.2, which encodes for the protein merlin.

Epidemiology
- NF1: incidence of 1 out of 3,000 live births with skin manifestations usually evident at birth.
- NF2: incidence of 1 out of 35,000 live births with typical onset of symptoms in late teens to early 20s.

Risk Factors
- With autosomal dominant transmission, a child has a 50% chance of inheriting the gene from an affected parent.

Clinical Features
- Cognitive impairment is one of the most common neurologic symptoms in children and adults. Intelligence quotient (IQ) is usually in the low-average range.
- Visual–spatial problems include impaired visual motor integration and impaired balance.
- Pain and gait abnormalities due to axonal sensorimotor polyneuropathy from neurofibromas on peripheral nerves, plexiform neurofibromas, or malignant peripheral nerve sheath tumors
- Paraplegia and tetraplegia due to spinal neurofibromas
- Neurogenic bladder and bowel
- Functional limitations may also result from bone abnormalities such as scoliosis and bone defects, leading to pseudoarthroses.
- Language and communication difficulties in NF2 patients due to facial weakness and hearing loss.

Diagnosis

Differential diagnosis
- NF1 and NF2
- Hereditary spinal neurofibromatosis
- Mosaic or segmental NF1
- Brain stem gliomas
- Cauda equina and conus medullaris syndromes
- Astrocytoma or meningioma

History
- NF1 children have skin changes such as café au lait spots evident at a young age (even at birth), freckling in the axillary or inguinal folds, and neurofibromas. Other diagnostic features include Lisch nodules (iris hamartomas), optic gliomas, and skeletal deformities.
  - Learning disabilities and attention deficit disorders
- NF2 patients present with hearing loss, balance impairments, vertigo due to vestibular schwannoma, and visual deficits from cataracts.
  - They have a predilection to multiple tumors, which include spinal cord gliomas, meningiomas, and schwannomas of the cranial or spinal nerves.

Treatment
- There is no cure for the disorder.
- NF1:
  - No treatment is needed for the Lisch nodules or café au lait spots. Patients who have significant disfigurement from large neurofibromas can have surgical removal of the tumors, but the tumors have a tendency to recur.
  - Tumors that cause pain, loss of function, or are rapidly growing can be removed.
  - Bracing for mild cases of scoliosis versus spinal fusion for rapid progression of dystrophic scoliosis
  - Consider bisphosphonates for pseudoarthroses and osteoporosis
  - Weight-bearing exercises to improve bone health
  - Chemotherapy versus radiation is considered for optic pathway gliomas.
- NF2:
  - Surgical resection of schwannomas
  - Chemotherapy for unresectable, progressive schwannomas or spinal cord schwannomas

– Resection of spinal cord tumors and/or radiosurgery for residual tumors or progressive disease
– Visual–spatial rehabilitation

Consultations
- Pediatric neurology
- Dermatology
- Otolaryngology
- Ophthalmology
- Genetics
- Physiatry
- Neurosurgery
- Orthopedics
- Plastic surgery
- Endocrinology
- Radiation oncology
- Radiology

Prognosis
- NF1: Variable clinical presentation with different manifestations among family members.
  – Most cases are mild and individuals have normal and productive lives.
  – Main concerns include disfigurement due to the cutaneous lesions.
  – Plexiform neurofibromas and malignant nerve sheath tumors can be difficult to resect and can lead to monoplegia, paraplegia, or tetraplegia. Malignant nerve sheath tumors are a significant cause of morbidity and mortality due to their difficulty to treat.

- NF2: Disease course is variable and can be progressive.
  – Vestibular schwannomas tend to grow slowly. Morbidity is due to impaired balance and hearing, which deteriorate over many years.
  – Studies have shown that younger age at diagnosis of NF2 is associated with decreased survival.
  – Schwannomatosis can also cause severe and disabling pain.
  – Damage to other cranial nerves and the brain stem can be life threatening.

Helpful Hints
- Most patients with NF1 can lead normal and productive lives, but are most concerned about their physical disfigurement.
- Patients with malignant peripheral nerve sheath tumors or recurrent spinal cord schwannomas have a complicated medical course and can require multiple surgeries for decompression, radiation, and/or chemotherapy, and may benefit from multiple inpatient rehabilitation stays to address their progressive functional deficits.

Suggested Readings
Hersh JH. Health supervision for children with neurofibromatosis. *Pediatrics.* 2008;121(3):633–642.

Patel CM, Ferner R, Grunfeld EA. A qualitative study of the impact of living with neurofibromatosis type 2. *Psychol Health Med.* 2011;16(1):19–28.

Williams VC, Lucas J, Babcock MA, et al. Neurofibromatosis type 1 revisited. *Pediatrics.* 2009;123(1):124–133.

Yohay K. Neurofibromatosis types 1 and 2. *Neurologist.* 2006;12(2):86–93.

Spinal Cord Compression

Rajesh R. Yadav MD

Description

Spinal cord compression (SCC) is a neurological emergency and if left untreated may result in permanent tetraplegia or paraplegia.

Etiology/Types

- Spinal cord impingement may occur with a primary spinal cord tumor or metastatic disease to the spine via direct tumor growth, spinal instability due to pathologic fracture, or vascular compromise.

Epidemiology

- SCC incidence in all patients with cancer is 5% to 10%.

Pathogenesis

- Development of spinal column compression with the affinity of tumor cells to the bone marrow in the spinal column is the first stage of metastatic epidural SCC.
- Enlargement of a spinal tumor mass anteriorly leads to impingement of the thecal sac and epidural venous plexus.
- Thoracic level is the most commonly affected by metastatic disease.
- With metastatic disease-related cortical bone destruction, vertebral body compression fracture and retropulsion of bony fragments can lead to epidural SCC.
- Tumor growth from the paraspinal region through the neural foramina can also lead to epidural SCC.
- Stenosis and obstruction of the epidural venous plexus and impaired venous and arterial circulation can lead to ischemic changes.
- Inflammatory mediators and edema further compromise the integrity of the spinal cord.

Risk Factors

- Cancers of the breast, lung, prostate, and kidney account for the majority of cancer SCC cases.
- Non-Hodgkin lymphoma and multiple myeloma account for 5% to 10% of neoplastic SCC cases.
- Primary spine tumors in the extradural space, including chordoma, chondrosarcoma, and vertebral hemangioma, account for 1% of all spinal tumors.
- Primary tumors such as astrocytoma and ependymoma make up 75% of all intrameduallary tumors.
- Examples of benign and primary intradural and extramedullary tumors include neurofibromas, schwannomas, and meningiomas.

Clinical Features

- Pain is a common symptom of a spinal tumor and is often worse in supine position.
- With spinal cord tumor, central pain may be present at or below the level of the tumor.
- Pain can be a major issue post treatment, including surgery, and may require the use of patient-controlled analgesia.
- In addition to the respiratory compromise due to neurological injury, pain may further interfere with normal breathing.
- Depending on the location and extent of SCC-related neurological decline, ability to perform basic activities of daily life (ADLs) and mobility are affected.
- With complete cord injury, flaccid and complete paralysis, loss of sensation, areflexia, and autonomic dysfunction are present below the level of injury.
- With injury at C5 or above, the respiratory muscles may be affected and ventilator may be needed.
- Flaccid paralysis may change to spastic paralysis over a period of days with hypertonia and increased deep tendon reflexes.
- With incomplete spinal cord injury, motor and sensory loss is incomplete and deep tendon reflexes may be hyperactive.
- With spinal shock, that is, spinal cord swelling, significant neurologic dysfunction may result and improvement may be noted over several days.
- Deficits depend on the level of injury and discrete syndromes may be present.
- With decreased activity, there is risk of deep venous thrombosis, contractures, pneumonia, pressure ulcers, and urinary tract infection.
- There may be inadequate emptying of bowel and bladder.
- With cauda equina injuries, lower extremities have hyporeflexic paralysis, often with pain and hyperesthesia in affected nerve distribution.
- With sacral and conus medullaris involvement, complete loss of bowel and bladder continence may occur.

Diagnosis

Differential diagnosis

- Mechanical low back pain with prior history of injury
- Chemotherapy-associated peripheral neuropathy leading to motor and sensory deficits
- Steroid myopathy leading to proximal weakness
- Brachial and lumbosacral plexopathy—neoplastic and/or post radiation
- Paraneoplastic syndrome
- Radiculopathy
- Radiation myelitis
- Transverse myelitis

History

- Back pain is the most frequent presenting symptom with 83% to 98% of patients experiencing axial or radicular back pain before diagnosis.
- Pain is often localized at the lesion site and tends to be progressive in severity over a period of time.
- Patients have difficulty sleeping owing to pain in a recumbent position.
- Spinal instability associated with vertebral body collapse can lead to mechanical back pain, which is exacerbated by movement.
- Neurologic deficits include:
  - Motor weakness—50% to 68% of patients are unable to ambulate at time of SCC diagnosis.
  - Sensory deficits (61%–78%)
  - Bowel or bladder deficits (57%–69%)
- Sudden or rapid progression of motor weakness.

Examination

- Motor weakness
- Sensory deficits
- Pain with palpation along spine
- Impaired reflexes, including deep tendon reflexes
- Clonus
- Pathologic upper motor neuron reflexes
- Decreased anal sphincter tone

Testing

- Spine MRI is the most reliable imaging modality for SCC diagnosis.
- PET scan to detect SCC may be helpful with unsuspected SCC.
- CT is crucial for neurosurgical interventions or radiation treatment.
- CT myelogram may be pursued in patients who cannot undergo MRI, such as patients with pacemakers or defibrillators.
- Bone scan may be useful in delineating the extent of osseous turnover, particularly with osteoblastic lesions. If spinal pathology is noted, particularly in symptomatic patients, more detailed imaging, including MRI and CT, should be considered.
- Plain spine radiographs for patients with back pain and cancer history can provide information about spinal alignment and instability.

Treatment

- Corticosteroids
  - Early initiation
  - Improved functional outcome despite no impact on survival times
  - Improvement in pain
- Radiation
  - Helps with:
    - Pain in 57% to 73% of patients
    - Recovery of motor function in 26% to 42%
    - Regaining ambulation in 26% to 35%
      - Less than 10% of patients who are completely paralyzed regain ambulation.
  - Indications include:
    - Radiosensitive tumors
    - Expected survival of 3 to 4 months
    - Inability to tolerate surgery
    - Total neurological deficit below level of spinal compression for more than 24 to 48 hours
    - Multilevel or diffuse disease
  - Treatment is often short term, although longer-term course is prescribed with multiple myeloma.
  - Can be given during rehabilitation efforts, including inpatient rehabilitation.
- Surgery
  - If patients can undergo surgery, they should.
  - Patients may not qualify for surgery if total neurological deficit below level of spinal compression has been present for more than 24 to 48 hours.
  - Interventions can include removal of metastatic lesion(s) via posterior and anterior approach, hardware placement, and use of methylmethacrylate and bone grafting.
  - Goals include:
    - Stabilization of spine
    - Decompression of spinal cord
    - Reduction of pain
    - Improvement in functional outcomes, including bowel, bladder, strength, and mobility
    - Minimizing orthotic use
  - Patients may need plastic surgery intervention for surgical defects.
    - May be more complicated in patients who have received radiation treatment previously
  - Patients may be appropriate for radiation treatment following surgery.

■ Rehabilitation
  - Improves function, quality of life, pain, and mood
  - Functional goals should be formulated in context of:
    • Functional deficits
    • Symptoms
    • Expected survival
    • Discharge plans
    • Further treatment plans
    • Patient and family expectations
  - Inpatient rehabilitation in SCC with metastatic cancer should be of shorter duration
  - Goals include:
    • Family training to allow for safe transfers and ADLs
    • Dispensing appropriate durable medical equipment
    • Management of neurogenic bowel and bladder

  • Symptom management, including pain
  • Assisting patient and family in coping with psychological distress
  • Teaching patient and family about skin care
  - Improvement in functional status may qualify patients for systemic treatment, including chemotherapy.
  - Use of indwelling catheter for neurogenic bladder may be a viable option in a patient with various symptoms, including fatigue, limited functional status, and poor prognosis.
  - Although laxatives and stool softeners are often needed owing to the use of opiates, nonpharmacologic interventions such as education, establishing time for elimination, use of warm liquids, and digital stimulation can also be helpful for neurogenic bowel management.

Table 15.1 Tokuhashi Scoring System

Characteristic	Score
General condition (performance status)	
Poor (PS 10%–40%)	0
Moderate (PS 50%–70%)	1
Good (PS 80%–100%)	2
No. of extraspinal bone metastases foci	
≥3	0
1–2	1
0	2
No. of metastases in the vertebral body	
≥3	0
2	1
1	2
Metastases to the major internal organs	
Unremovable	0
Removable	1
No metastases	2
Primary site of the cancer	
Lung, osteosarcoma, stomach, bladder, esophagus, pancreas	0
Liver, gallbladder, unidentified	1
Others	2
Kidney, uterus	3
Rectum	4
Thyroid, breast, prostate, carcinoid tumor	5
Palsy	
Complete (Frankel A, B)	0
Incomplete (Frankel C, D)	1
None (Frankel E)	2

Total Score

0–8 → **Conservative treatment**
Predicted prognosis 6 months >

9–11 → **Palliative surgery**
Predicted prognosis 6 months ≤
  • Single lesion
  • No metastases to the major internal organs

12–15 → **Excisional surgery**
Predicted prognosis 1 year ≤

Criteria of predicted prognosis: Total Score (TS) 0–8 = >6 mo; TS 9–11 = ≤6 mo; TS 12–15 = ≤ 1 yr

Source: www.jkma.org/ArticleImage/1119JKMA/jkma-49-1097-i004-l.jpg

II: Primary Concerns or Conditions

Prognosis

- Functional prognosis is better in patients who present earlier and are ambulatory.
- The median survival varies but frequently can be from 2 to 6 months.
- Ambulatory patients after treatment have a longer median survival (7.9 months) than nonambulatory patients (1.2 months).
- More favorable prognosis is seen with primary cancers, including myeloma, breast, and prostate.
  - Single compression site and hemoglobin level of more than 12 g/dL with metastatic prostate SCC are also good prognostic factors.
- Patients with gastrointestinal and lung cancers can have shorter survival time (less than 3 months) than breast and genitourinary cancers (3–5 months).
- The Tokuhashi scoring system may be useful in survival prognostication with parameters including general condition, number of spinal/extraspinal metastases, primary site of the cancer, and severity of spinal cord injury (see Table 15.1).

Helpful Hints

- In a patient with a history of cancer, new or worsening back pain should be investigated aggressively.
- Pain may occur months prior to neurologic decline.
- Sudden or rapid neurologic decline is a neurosurgical emergency.
- Rehabilitation of SCC in cancer patients can be affected by metastatic osseous disease in the limbs (i.e., weight-bearing and range-of-motion restrictions may be necessary).

Suggested Readings

Abrahm J, Banffy MB, Harris MB. Spinal cord compression in patients with advanced metastatic cancer "all I care about is walking and living my life". *JAMA.* 2008;299(8):937–946.

Byrne TN, Borges LF, Loeffler JS. Metastatic epidural spinal cord compression: Update on management. *Semin Oncol.* 2006;33:307–311.

Guo Y, Young B, Palmer JL, et al. Prognostic factors for survival in metastatic spinal cord compression: A retrospective study in a rehabilitation setting. *Am J Phys Med Rehabil.* 2003;82:665–668.

Shiue K, Sahgal A, Chow E, et al. Management of metastatic spinal cord compression. *Expert Rev Anticancer Ther.* 2010;10(5):697–708.

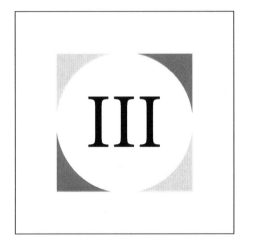

Cancer- or Treatment-Related Symptoms

Anemia

Etsuko Aoki MD PhD

Description

Anemia is commonly seen in patients with cancer. It is often related to antineoplastic therapies and/or disease progression. Anemia is a frequent cause of fatigue in cancer patients. Fatigue is a frequent cause of reduced quality of life (QOL).

Anemia is defined as follows:

- Mild: hemoglobin (Hgb) 10 g/dL—lower limit of normal
- Moderate: Hgb 8.0 to 9.9 g/dL
- Severe: Hgb 6.5 to 7.9 g/dL
- Life threatening: Hgb lower than 6.5 g/dL

Etiology/Types

Anemia can occur due to (a) direct effects of cancer, (b) effects of the products of neoplasms, or (c) effects of antineoplastic therapy. More than one contributor can be present.

- Direct effects of cancer:
  - External bleeding (gastrointestinal (GI) or genitourinary (GU) cancer)
  - Impaired iron absorption (GI cancer)
  - Internal bleeding (liver, spleen, retroperitoneal, ovarian cancer)
  - Hemophagocytosis (leukemia, T-cell lymphoma)
  - Bone marrow replacement by tumor cells
- Effects of the products of neoplasms:
  - Autoimmune hemolysis (chronic lymphocytic leukemia)
  - Microangiopathic hemolysis
  - Pure red-cell aplasia (hematologic malignancies)
  - Anemia of chronic inflammation
  - Amyloidosis (multiple myeloma)
- Effects of antineoplastic therapy:
  - Chemotherapy
  - Radiation therapy causing bone marrow suppression

Epidemiology

- The most frequent hematological manifestation in patients with cancer
- In a prospective study from The European Cancer Anemia Survey, 40% of patients with cancer had an Hgb of lower than 12 g/dL at initiation of treatment and 75% of patients who received chemotherapy developed anemia within 6 months.

Pathogenesis

- Three categories should be considered:
  - Red blood cell (RBC) loss from the body
  - Increased RBC destruction: hemolysis
  - Decreased RBC production in the bone marrow

Risk Factors

- Low baseline Hgb level
- Site of primary tumor, including leukemia, multiple myeloma, and lymphoma
- Platinum-containing chemotherapy regimen
- Female gender
- Advanced age
- Poor performance status

Diagnosis

History

- Fatigue
- Dyspnea on exertion, dyspnea at rest (more advanced)
- Palpitation, "roaring in the ears" secondary to decreased blood pressure
- Symptoms of volume depletion (muscle cramps, postural dizziness, syncope)
- Cardiac complications (angina, myocardial infarction, arrhythmia, congestive heart failure)

Examination

- Pallor
- Anemic conjunctivae
- Tachycardia, arrhythmia
- Jaundice (hemolysis).
- Bone tenderness (bone marrow infiltration)
- Hepatosplenomegaly
- Lymphadenopathy

Testing

- Complete blood counts (CBC) with mean corpuscular volume (MCV), mean corpuscular hemoglobin (MCH), mean corpuscular hemoglobin concentration, (MCHC), reticulocyte count, and white blood cell (WBC) differentiation
- Peripheral blood smear
- Iron study, serum folic acid, vitamin B_{12} level
- Total bilirubin, lactate dehydrogenase (LDH), haptoglobin
- Bone marrow examination

Functional impact
- Fatigue
- Reduced tolerability of daily activities
- Reduced QOL

Treatment
- If nutritional deficiency (iron, vitamin B$_{12}$, or folic acid) exists, replete.
- Target Hgb is generally 7 to 9 g/dL. If patient has cardiopulmonary symptoms, consider transfusion to maintain higher Hgb level.
- If Hgb is equal to or less than 7 g/dL, transfuse RBC to bring Hgb up to approximately 10 g/dL.
- If Hgb is 7 to 9 g/dL with symptoms, transfuse RBC to bring Hgb up to approximately 10 g/dL or consider the use of erythropoietin stimulating agents (ESAs).
- Transfusion versus ESAs: Transfusion can rapidly ameliorate symptoms related to anemia, whereas with ESAs a meaningful response will be expected in weeks to months. ESAs are related to thromboembolic risk and offer questionable improved survival in patients with anemia owing to myelosuppressive chemotherapy.
- ESAs are *not indicated* for anemia unrelated to chemotherapy (except in patients with lower-risk myelodysplastic syndrome to avoid transfusions).
- ESAs are *not indicated* for anemia in patients receiving myelosuppressive chemotherapy for curative intent.
- ESAs are *not indicated* for anemia in patients receiving radiation therapy alone.

Prognosis
- Anemia has been linked to adverse prognosis in some malignancies (owing to reduced oxygenation that can lead to poorer response to chemotherapy or radiation therapy).

Helpful Hint
- Monitor CBC and fatigue level, especially in patients receiving chemotherapy.

Suggested Readings
Calabrich A, Kats A. Management of anemia in cancer patients. *Future Oncol.* 2011;7:507–517.

Hinkel JM, Li EC, Sherman SL. Insights and perspectives in the clinical operational management of cancer-related anemia. *JNCCN.* 2010;8:S38–S55.

Stasi R, Abriani L, Beccaglia P, et al. Cancer-related fatigue. *Cancer.* 2003;98:1786–1798.

III: Cancer- or Treatment-Related Symptoms

Anorexia–Cachexia

Julio Silvestre MD ▪ Rony Dev DO

Background

Anorexia, the loss of appetite and reduced caloric intake, is common among patients with chronic illness, including infections, chronic pain, and cancer. Anorexia may result in *cachexia*—involuntary weight loss—a hypermetabolic state characterized by progressive sarcopenia (loss of skeletal muscle), with or without loss of fat. Unlike starvation, cachexia is not reversed by increasing caloric intake. Cancer anorexia–cachexia syndrome severely reduces patients' quality of life.

Epidemiology

- 60% to 80% of patients with advanced cancer have anorexia in the last year of life. Anorexia may be accompanied with nausea, which can result in physical discomfort.

Pathogenesis

- Increased caloric intake is dependent on the palatability of food, which is controlled by the cranial nerves, including the olfactory, glossopharyngeal, and facial nerves.
- The feeling of satiety is mediated by the autonomic sensory nerves innervating the proximal gastrointestinal tract and contained in the afferent arm of the vagus nerve, which influence the hypothalamic areas responsible for feeding.
- Other factors that control appetite include neurotransmitters (serotonin, dopamine, and histamine), ghrelin and leptin, corticotropin releasing factor, neuropeptide Y, and alpha-melanocyte-stimulating hormone.

Risk Factors

- Drugs that result in anorexia include: selective serotonin reuptake inhibitors, amphetamines, methylphenidate, stimulants (caffeine, nicotine, and cocaine), and opiates (result in gastroparesis).
- Chronic pain
- Zinc deficiency
- Anxiety disorders and depression

Diagnosis

The symptom of anorexia is nonspecific and may be associated with endocrine, gastrointestinal, renal, pulmonary, immune, neurological, psychiatric, and other medical disorders.

Visual, numerical, and verbal rating scales have been developed to measure the subjective symptom of anorexia. The Edmonton Symptom Assessment Scale is one method often used and ranks symptoms on a numerical scale from 0 to 10. See Figure 17.1 and Tables 17.1 and 17.2.

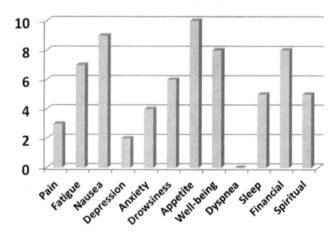

Figure 17.1 ESAS with significant anorexia—appetite is rated as 10.

History and examination

- Alterations in taste and smell
- Xerostomia or oral dryness
- Dysphagia

Testing

- Diet diary assesses caloric intake
- Body mass index (body mass divided by the square of patient's height)
- Dual-energy x-ray absorptiometry or bioelectrical impedance analysis measures body composition

Treatment

Medical

- For xerostomia, frequent oral hygiene, rinsing in cold water, sucking on ice chips, and chewing sugarless gum may improve salivation and provide comfort.
- For decreased taste, a short-term trial of zinc supplementation may help.

Table 17.1   Edmonton Symptom Assessment System—Revised

Please circle the number that best describes how you feel NOW:

No Pain	0	1	2	3	4	5	6	7	8	9	10	Worst Possible Pain
No Tiredness (*Tiredness = lack of energy*)	0	1	2	3	4	5	6	7	8	9	10	Worst Possible Tiredness
No Drowsiness (*Drowsiness = feeling sleepy*)	0	1	2	3	4	5	6	7	8	9	10	Worst Possible Drowsiness
No Nausea	0	1	2	3	4	5	6	7	8	9	10	Worst Possible Nausea
No Lack of Appetite	0	1	2	3	4	5	6	7	8	9	10	Worst Possible Lack of Appetite
No Shortness of Breath	0	1	2	3	4	5	6	7	8	9	10	Worst Possible Shortness of Breath
No Depression (*Depression = feeling sad*)	0	1	2	3	4	5	6	7	8	9	10	Worst Possible Depression
No Anxiety (*Anxiety = feeling nervous*)	0	1	2	3	4	5	6	7	8	9	10	Worst Possible Anxiety
Best Well-Being (*Well-being = how you feel overall*)	0	1	2	3	4	5	6	7	8	9	10	Worst Possible Well-Being
No _____ Other Problem (*for example, constipation*)	0	1	2	3	4	5	6	7	8	9	10	Worst Possible _____

Source: Reprinted from Watanabe S. A multicenter study comparing two numerical versions of the Edmonton Symptom Assessments System in Palliative Care Patients. *J Pain Symptom Manage*, 2011;41(2):456–468. Reprinted with permission from Elsevier.

III: Cancer- or Treatment-Related Symptoms

Table 17.2   ESAS With Significant Anorexia—Appetite Is Rated as 10

Pain	10
Fatigue	9
Nausea	0
Depression	1
Anxiety	5
Drowsiness	3
Appetite	10
Well-being	4
Dyspnea	0
Sleep	5

- Corticosteroid therapy and megestrol acetate have been shown to improve appetite and lead to modest weight gain.
- A randomized trial comparing the effects of cannabis extract, tetrahydrocannabinol, and placebo reported no significant difference in appetite, nor in quality of life in cancer patients but may be helpful in patients with HIV.

Counseling
- Emphasis is on the pleasure and social benefits of eating with the family over the nutritional intake.

Complications of treatment
- Megestrol acetate may cause side effects such as thromboembolism, adrenal insufficiency, and low testosterone in male patients.

Helpful Hint
- Initial treatment of anorexia–cachexia syndrome should focus on treating symptoms such as uncontrolled pain, constipation, and mood abnormalities.

Suggested Readings

Berenstein EG, Ortiz Z. Megestrol acetate for the treatment of anorexia-cachexia syndrome. *Cochrane Database Syst Rev.* 2005;18(2):CD004310.

Del Fabbro, Hui D, Dalal S, et al. Clinical outcomes and contributors to weight loss in a cancer cachexia clinic. *J Palliat Med.* 2011;14(9):1004–1008.

Fearon K, Strasser F, Anker SD, et al. Definition and classification of cancer cachexia: An international consensus. *Lancet Oncol.* 2011;12:489–495.

Asthenia

Ying Guo MD MS

Description

Asthenia in cancer patients can have two components: general weakness and a decrease in exercise tolerance.

Etiology

- General weakness can be due to:
  - Muscle wasting
  - Disuse atrophy
  - Malnutrition
- Poor exercise tolerance can be due to dysfunction in other than the musculoskeletal system, such as:
  - Anemia
  - Cardiac comorbidity
  - Pulmonary complications

Epidemiology

- 40% to 50% of cancer patients referred for inpatient rehabilitation have asthenia.

Pathogenesis

- Cancer-related muscle loss, or cachexia, is the cause of death for approximately 2 million people worldwide and severely reduces quality of life.
- Cachexia is associated with cytokines such as tumor necrosis factor-alpha, which can trigger degradatory pathways through nuclear factor-kappa B signaling and activate the ubiquitin-proteasome system causing muscle proteolysis.

Risk Factors

- Weight loss
- Prolonged hospital stay or bed rest
- Cardiac and pulmonary comorbidity
- Older age

Clinical Features

- Difficulty with transfers and ambulation; usually, functional score for both activities is at moderate assistance or better with decreased tolerance for therapy activities.
- Can also coexist with anorexia, anemia, malnutrition, depression, and other conditions
- Decreased balance, increased risk for falls

Diagnosis

Differential diagnosis

- Steroid myopathy: patients with myopathy are usually on steroids, and weakness is more profound at the hip flexors and extensors. With tapering of steroids, function usually improves significantly and quickly.
- Metastatic spinal cord compression: usually has sudden onset, sensory loss, bowel/bladder dysfunction. This is a medical emergency.

History

- Gradual onset, usually after a prolonged illness
- Progressive disability and worsening performance status
- This worsening-performance status may impact the patient's ability to receive further treatment for cancer.

Examination

- Muscle strength is usually better than 3/5 in all four extremities.

Treatment

- Increase sitting time so patient can improve his or her endurance, trunk strength, and tolerate upright positioning.
- Address other medical conditions simultaneously, such as anemia, malnutrition, sleep, pain, and mood disorders.
- Progressively increase exercise dose and duration
- Teach patient fatigue management.
- Balance training

Prognosis

- Short-term inpatient rehabilitation is effective in improving functional status.
- Outpatient therapy is effective in maintaining functional level.
- Patients' function will likely deteriorate as disease progresses.
- If left untreated, patient is likely to get weaker.

Helpful Hint

■ All cancer patients can benefit from some level of rehabilitation and restoration of their function. Due to the chronic nature of cancer, which renders multiple insults (including chemotherapy, radiation, and surgery), patients should build up their functional status in-between treatments.

Suggested Readings

Cole RP, Scialla SJ, Bednarz L. Functional recovery in cancer rehabilitation. *Arch Phys Med Rehabil.* 2000;81:623–627.

Guo Y, Palmer JL, Kaur G, et al. Nutritional status of cancer patients and its relationship to function in an inpatient rehabilitation setting. *Support Care Cancer.* 2005;13:169–175.

Guo Y, Persyn L, Palmer JL, Bruera E. Incidence of and risk factors for transferring cancer patients from rehabilitation to acute care units. *Am J Phys Med Rehabil.* 2008;87:647–653.

Autonomic Nervous System Dysfunction

Ying Guo MD MS

Description

Autonomous nervous dysfunction in cancer patients can lead to symptoms such as fatigue, cachexia, anorexia, bowel and bladder dysfunction, and orthostatic hypotension. It can also adversely impact survival.

Etiology/Types

- Paraneoplastic systemic autonomic neuropathy
- Chemotherapy-induced peripheral polyneuropathy
- Bed rest, lack of exercise
- Malnutrition

Epidemiology

- About 80% of patients with advanced cancer have autonomic dysfunction (AD). AD has been described in patients with:
  - Bronchogenic carcinoma
  - Lymphoma
  - Leukemia
  - Pancreatic cancer
  - Prostate cancer
  - Breast cancer
  - Ovarian cancer
  - Testicular cancer

Pathogenesis

In the cancer patient, it is hypothesized that:

- Sympathetic fiber activity increases, possibly promoting metastasis
- Parasympathetic activity decreases, causing anorexia, cachexia, insomnia, bladder and bowel dysfunction, poor sense of well-being, depression, and anxiety.

Risk Factors

- Diabetes mellitus or other comorbidity-causing neuropathy
- Prolonged hospital stay, bed rest, lack of activity
- Older age

Clinical Features

- Difficulty with ambulation
- Decreased tolerance for therapy activities
- Can coexist with anorexia, anemia, malnutrition, depression, and other conditions
- Falls-related injury

Diagnosis

History

- When a patient has orthostatic hypotension, early satiety, constipation, erectile dysfunction, anorexia, fatigue, or cachexia, one should have a high suspicion of autonomic nervous system (ANS) dysfunction.
- Increase in patient's fall risk, decrease in performance status
- Can impact the patient's ability to receive further treatment for cancer

Tests

- Quantitative sudomotor axon reflex test (QSART), quantitative test of sudomotor function
- The composite autonomic scoring scale (CASS), which includes QSART, orthostatic blood pressure, heart rate response to tilt, heart rate response to deep breathing, the Valsalva ratio, beat-to-beat blood pressure (BP) measurements during phases II and IV of the Valsalva maneuver, tilt, and deep breathing, provides a useful 10-point scale of autonomic function.
- Heart rate variability test, which provides indices for both parasympathetic and sympathetic autonomic function

Treatment

Medical

- Increase sitting tolerance. Start with sitting at the edge of the bed 3× per day for meals; gradually progress to a total of 3 hours per episode, 3× per day in chair. This simple intervention can prevent aspiration pneumonia, and improve patient's endurance, trunk strength, and tolerance for upright posture.
- Treatment of orthostatic hypotension with medication
- Other medical conditions should be treated simultaneously, including anemia, dehydration, malnutrition, sleep, pain, and mood disorders.
- Activities that increase vagal nerve activity: relaxation, meditation, massage, guided imagery, yoga, deep breathing, acupuncture

Therapy/rehabilitation

- Lower extremity large muscle group activation prior to functional activities such as step in place
- Increase overall muscle tone

III: Cancer- or Treatment-Related Symptoms

49

- Exercise dose and duration should be increased progressively.
- Fatigue management
- Compression stockings, abdominal binder to prevent drastic blood pressure drop and related symptoms of dizziness and loss of consciousness
- Hydration during therapy
- Frequent rest
- Short-term inpatient rehabilitation can effectively reverse orthostatic hypotension in many patients.

Prognosis

- Patient's function will likely deteriorate as disease progresses.
- If left untreated, patient is likely to get worse.
- Low heart rate variability is associated with shorter survival.

Helpful Hints

- Recognize symptoms early.
- Treating symptoms can improve quality of life.
- Promote parasympathetic function and reduce sympathetic tone.

Suggested Readings

Bruera E, Chadwick S, Fox R, et al. Study of cardiovascular autonomic insufficiency in advanced cancer patients. *Cancer Treat Rep.* 1986;70:1383–1387.

Ewing DJ, Martyn CN, Young RJ, Clarke BF. The value of cardiovascular autonomic function tests: 10 years experience in diabetes. *Diabetes Care.* 1985;8:491–498.

Strasser F, Palmer JL, Schover LR, et al. The impact of hypogonadism and autonomic dysfunction on fatigue, emotional function, and sexual desire in male patients with advanced cancer: A pilot study. *Cancer.* 2006;107:2949–2957.

Walsh D, Nelson KA. Autonomic nervous system dysfunction in advanced cancer. *Support Care Cancer.* 2002;10:523–528.

Chemotherapy: Cardiomyopathy

Peter Kim MD

Description

Cardiotoxicity, and in particular, the development of heart failure, is a known chemotherapy-related side effect. Chemotherapy-induced cardiomyopathy is the development of heart failure after the administration of chemotherapeutic agents.

Etiology

- The most common groups of agents that cause heart failure are:
  - Anthracyclines
  - Alkylating agents
  - Monoclonal antibody-based tyrosine kinase inhibitors

Epidemiology

- The incidence of heart failure depends on the agent used, cumulative dose, administration schedule, and preexisting heart disease.
- The incidence ranges from 0.5% to 28%. The most common agents are:
  - Doxorubicin   3% to 26%
  - Cyclophosphamide   7% to 28%
  - Trastuzumab   2% to 28%

Pathogenesis

- The pathogenesis has not been completely defined, and each chemotherapeutic agent has its own particular mechanism of action.
- The common final pathway for each agent is likely related to disturbances in the end-signaling pathways of the heart that affect myocyte contractility, hypertrophy, and cell death via free radical formation or direct enodothelial injury.

Risk Factors

- Increasing cumulative dose of chemotherapy
- Faster rate of administration
- Younger or older age
- Preexisting cardiac disease, such as coronary artery disease and congestive heart failure
- Mediastinal radiation exposure:
  - Exposure to as low as 30 gray (Gy) has been linked to myocardial fibrosis, development of pericardial effusions, and coronary artery disease.

Clinical Features

Patients can present acutely or subacutely with blood pressure changes, thrombosis, ventricular or junctional arrhythmias, left ventricular failure, pericarditis, or myocarditis.

Chronic cardiotoxicity can result in progressive systolic ventricular dysfunction.

Diagnosis

Differential diagnosis

- Chronic obstructive pulmonary disorder (COPD) exacerbation
- Acute coronary syndromes
- Pulmonary embolism
- Malignant pleural or pericardial effusion

History

- Dyspnea on exertion, paroxysmal nocturnal dyspnea, orthopnea
- Persistent cough or wheezing
- Increasing abdominal girth
- Palpitations or irregular heart rhythm

Examination

- Elevated jugular venous pressure
- S_3 heard on cardiac auscultation
- Pulmonary rales
- Lower-extremity edema

Testing

- EKG to rule out arrhythmia
- Chest x-ray to rule out congestive heart failure
- Brain natriuretic peptide level to assess for left ventricular dysfunction
- Echocardiogram:
  - No consensus guideline in regard to the appropriate frequency of echocardiogram studies.
  - General principle is to check before receiving the initial cycle and after each subsequent cycle.
  - Symptoms of heart failure should prompt repeat testing.

- Radionucleotide ventriculography (RNV)/multigated acquisition scan (MUGA):
  - May be used as an alternative to an echocardiogram to monitor left heart function.
- Coronary angiogram to exclude ischemic heart disease

Treatment

Medical options
- Treatment of symptomatic heart failure—diuretic, angiotensin-converting enzyme (ACE) inhibitor, beta-blocker
- Cardiac risk factor reduction
- Discontinuation of chemotherapeutic agent

Surgery
- Synchronized pacing, ventricular assist devices, cardiac transplantation

Exercise
- An individualized approach to exercise is recommended. Low- to moderate-intensity exercise training programs have been shown to be beneficial in chronic stable heart failure.
- Heart rate-derived exercise may be inaccurate owing to medical therapy and loss of chronotropic reserve.
- Oxygen consumption measurements (peak VO_2) can offer objective assessment of functional capacity.

Prognosis
- Prompt diagnosis of chemotherapy-related cardiomyopathy is key. If undiagnosed or untreated, 10-year mortality can be as high as 75%.
- Dependent on the chemotherapeutic agent
  - Anthracycline-related cardiotoxicity is frequently not reversible.
  - 80% of patients with trastuzumab cardiotoxicity shown to have improvement with treatment.

Helpful Hints
- Prevention is the best way for avoiding chemotherapy-induced cardiomyopathy. Patients should be monitored closely with serial echocardiograms while undergoing treatment.
- If patients do develop chemotherapy-induced cardiomyopathy, they should be started on a standard heart failure regimen with an ACE inhibitor and beta-blocker.

Suggested Readings

Ewer MS, Yeh ET. *Cancer and the Heart*. Hamilton, Ontario: BC Decker; 2006.

Gharib MI, Burnett AK. Chemotherapy-induced cardiotoxicity: Current practice and prospects of prophylaxis. *Eur J Heart Fail*. 2002;4:235–242.

Pina IL, Apstein CS, Balady, GJ, et al. Exercise and heart failure. AHA Scientific Statement. *Circulation*. 2003; 107:1210–1225.

Yeh ET, Bickford CL. Cardiovascular complications of cancer therapy. *JACC*. 2009;53:2231–2247.

Chemotherapy: Chemobrain

Arash Asher MD

Description
Cognitive changes after cancer or cancer treatment, commonly referred to as "chemobrain," have become an increasing concern for cancer patients and survivors. Treatments for noncentral nervous system (CNS) tumors can cause both temporary and long-term cognitive changes that can significantly impact quality of life and occupational goals.

Etiology/Types
- Neurotoxicity from chemotherapy is one obvious hypothesis, hence the colloquial term "chemobrain."
- However, many other factors may affect cognition in cancer patients, including radiation therapy, anesthesia from surgery, genetic factors, depression, anxiety, sleep dysfunction, hormonal changes, cancer-related fatigue, inactivity, nutritional changes, and so forth. Therefore, "chemobrain" may not be the most accurate term for this clinical problem.

Epidemiology
- Up to 75% of cancer patients experience cognitive changes during treatment.
- 20% to 30% of cancer patients continue to experience cognitive changes after cancer treatment.

Pathogenesis
- Immune dysfunction and an altered cytokine profile are proposed etiologies.
- Direct neurotoxic effects of cancer treatment, oxidative damage, microemboli, and genetic predisposition may also play a role.

Risk Factors
- Young cancer patients may be more significantly affected by cognitive changes.
- Genetic predisposition, including APO-epsilon-4
- Certain chemotherapy may be especially neurotoxic, such as 5-fluorouracil, methotrexate.

Clinical Features
- Symptoms are typically subtle but may be very troubling to the patient.
- Difficulty with multitasking and executive function
- Difficulty with word retrieval and naming
- Poor short-term memory
- Difficulty with concentration or attention
- Slower processing speeds
- Long-term memories are spared
- Personal relationships, return to work, self-confidence, and community reintegration can be affected by cognitive changes after cancer treatment.

Diagnosis
Differential diagnosis
- Mood disorders, such as anxiety or depression
- Other cognitive disorders such as early dementia

History
- Cognitive symptoms follow, not precede, chemotherapy administration.

Examination
- Neurological exam should be normal and nonfocal.

Testing
- Subjective evaluations and self-assessment tools can be useful screening tools (i.e., The Functional Assessment of Cancer Therapy–Cognitive Function Scale).
- Neuropsychological testing can be very useful in identifying deficits in a variety of cognitive domains, including executive functioning, memory, processing speed, visuospatial skills, language, and emotional state.
- Imaging of the brain can rule out other factors, such as metastatic disease, if indicated.

Treatment
- Coexisting and contributing problems, such as sleep dysfunction, anxiety, depression, cancer-related fatigue, hot flashes, and so forth, should be managed.
- Compensatory strategies: time management, use of calendars and other memory aids, alteration of work environment, vocational retraining
- Possible trial of stimulants, such as methylphenidate or modafinil

III: Cancer- or Treatment-Related Symptoms

Prognosis

■ 80% return to baseline cognitive functioning within 6 to 9 months after completion of cancer therapy.

■ 20% to 25% may continue to have cognitive changes.

Helpful Hint

■ Exercise has not yet been evaluated as a tool for cognitive dysfunction among cancer patients although there is good evidence that it improves cognition among older adults. Given the many other benefits of exercise for cancer survivors, it should be recommended to all cancer patients.

Suggested Readings

Ahles TA, Root JC, Ryan EL. Cancer- and cancer treatment-associated cognitive change: An update on the state of the science. *J Clin Oncol.* 2012;30(30):3675–3686.

Asher A. Cognitive dysfunction among cancer survivors. *Am J Phys Med Rehabil.* 2011;90(5 suppl 1):S16–S26.

Chemotherapy: Peripheral Neuropathy

Ying Guo MD MS

Description

Peripheral polyneuropathy caused by neurotoxic agents affecting the sensory, motor, and autonomic nervous systems

Etiology/Types

- The main chemotherapy agents that cause peripheral neuropathy are:
  - Platinum agents
  - Taxanes
  - Vinca alkaloids
  - Thalidomide
  - Bortezomib
  - Ixabepilone

Epidemiology

- Chemotherapy-induced peripheral neuropathy (CIPN) commonly occurs in 30% to 40% of patients, but its incidence can vary from 0% to 70%.

Pathogenesis

- Chemotoxins can interfere with microtubule-based function in the axons (vinca alkaloids, taxanes, ixabepilone). This type of neuropathy can be reversible.
- Axonal loss (thalidomide)
- Apoptosis of the dorsal root ganglion (platinum agents)

Risk Factors

- Chemotherapeutic agent, longer duration of therapy, higher cumulative dose
- Concomitant use of other neurotoxic agents
- Advanced age
- Diabetes
- Alcohol use
- Other types of neuropathy
- Genetic

Clinical Features

- Paresthesias and pain in sensory neuropathies
- Symptoms often start in the fingers and toes and spread proximally in a "glove and stocking" distribution
- CIPN can begin weeks to months after initial treatment.
- Severe case can present with ataxia and gait abnormality.
- Decreased sensation in the hands leads to impairment of activities of daily living.
- Difficulty with balance and ataxia causes increased fall risk, especially when vision is compromised, such as in the shower, in the dark, and so forth.
- Pain can also cause limitation in function.

Diagnosis

Differential diagnosis

- Critical care neuropathy
- Diabetic neuropathy
- ETOH (ethanol)-induced neuropathy
- Myopathy

History

- Gradual onset, may not be reversible
- Can start many months after the initiation of chemotherapy
- Lower extremities may have more severe symptoms

Examination

- Decreased sensation
- Allodynia, hyperesthesia
- Difficulty with balance and ataxia in severe cases

Testing

- Electrodiagnostic studies will be able to provide information on sensory and motor nerve function.
- Quantitative sensory studies can provide information on small fibers.

Treatment

- Symptom treatment:
  - Selective serotonin reuptake inhibitor/serotonin-norepinephrine reuptake inhibitor
  - Gabapentin/pregabalin
  - Tricyclic antidepressants
  - Opioids
  - Topical agents: lidocaine, anti-inflammatory drugs
- Integrative treatment
  - Acupuncture
  - Nerve stimulation
  - Behavior intervention
  - Desensitization
  - Orthotics
  - Adaptive equipment

III: Cancer- or Treatment-Related Symptoms

55

Prognosis

- Can depend on the agent and duration of administration. Platinum-induced peripheral neuropathy may not be reversible.

Helpful Hints

- Should inform oncologist with early symptoms. Chemotherapy dose reduction or delay may decrease disability.
- Monitor the patient's functional status and render therapy, orthotics, and adaptive equipment as needed.

Suggested Readings

Dietrich J, Wen PY. Neurologic complications of chemotherapy. In: Schiff D, Kesari S, Wen PY, eds. *Cancer Neurology in Clinical Practice*. 2nd ed. Totowa, NJ: Humana Press; 2008:287.

Schiff D, Wen PY, van den Bent MJ. Neurological adverse effects caused by cytotoxic and targeted therapies. *Nat Rev Clin Oncol*. 2009;6:596.

Sioka C, Kyritsis AP. Central and peripheral nervous system toxicity of common chemotherapeutic agents. *Cancer Chemother Pharmacol*. 2009;63:761.

Cognitive Dysfunction

Jennie L. Rexer PhD ABPP-CN

Description

Cognitive dysfunction is common in cancer patients. It can be due to the disease itself or as a result of treatment.

Etiology/Types

- Cognitive dysfunction is common in neurooncology patients, and is often the presenting symptom in brain tumor patients. The course is usually related to tumor momentum and disease progression.
- Cognitive dysfunction can also be present in noncentral nervous system (non-CNS) cancers owing to a wide range of etiologies, including metabolic and neuroendocrine factors, side effects such as anemia, fatigue, pain, mood, and also treatment effects.
- Chemotherapy, hormonal therapy, and immunotherapy can all cause cognitive side effects. It has long been recognized that cancer patients report reduced cognitive efficiency during treatment, but in the past this was assumed to be associated with nonneurologic factors such as stress or depression. Only recently have some of the neurobiological bases of cognitive dysfunction been revealed.
- Cognitive difficulties associated with chemotherapy can be acute, owing to neurotoxicity or direct injury to parenchyma, as well as other reasons.
- Cognitive difficulties associated with both chemotherapy and cranial radiation can also be delayed, and progressive, owing to injury to progenitor cells, myelin damage, and cerebral atrophy, among others.
- The great majority of patients with chemotherapy-related mild cognitive dysfunction will have returned to baseline in approximately 1 year. However, there is evidence that a minority of patients will experience persistent cognitive difficulties.

Epidemiology

- Cognitive impairment is the most common neurologic problem associated with brain tumors and is evident at the time of diagnosis in 50% to 80% of patients.

- The incidence of cognitive impairment associated with non-CNS cancers and treatment effects is variable.

Risk Factors

- Age
- Exposure to high doses of chemotherapy, or high levels of cranial radiation
- Intrathecal administration of chemotherapy
- The role of genetics in vulnerability to cognitive symptoms at this point is not clear

Clinical Features

- In brain tumor patients, deficits are more variable and less severe than those associated with sudden onset neurologic events, such as stroke.
- The severity and type of cognitive deficits can be related to tumor location, size, and rate of progression.
- Impairments in attention/concentration, memory, cognitive–motor processing speed, and executive abilities are not uncommon.
- Neurobehavioral symptoms, such as apathy/reduced initiation, impulsivity, and impaired insight may also be present.
- Clinical features of cognitive dysfunction in non-CNS cancer patients are extremely variable.
- Cognitive difficulties in patients reporting chemotherapy-related mild cognitive impairment are also quite variable, though the presence of mildly reduced learning and retrieval on memory testing, as well as mildly reduced divided attention (such as "multitasking"), are common.
- Patients with neurocognitive symptoms may have difficulty attending to and learning rehabilitation strategies, and there may be little carry over from one rehabilitation session to the next.
- Similarly, patients with cognitive difficulties may have difficulty learning at-home treatment such as wound care, use of prosthetics, and so forth, and may have difficulty remembering to take their medications, among other potential problems.

III: Cancer- or Treatment-Related Symptoms

■ Patients with poor insight into their cognitive difficulties may not see the need for rehabilitation nor for safety precautions.

Diagnosis

Differential diagnosis
■ Preexisting intellectual or other cognitive difficulties
■ Dementia
■ Mood disturbance

Neuropsychological evaluation
Neuropsychological evaluation is a standardized method for assessing the type, degree, and course of cognitive dysfunction. These results are important for making safety recommendations, such as a patient's ability to live independently, manage medications and finances, drive, and return to work or school. Neuropsychological evaluations are often used in capacity and disability evaluations. Results can be used for discharge planning, to tailor treatment recommendations, and to help maximize compliance. Neuropsychological testing is particularly useful for distinguishing between neurological and psychological factors, as well as the degree of overlap.

■ Examination should involve major cognitive domains, including:
  – Attention
  – Memory
  – Visuospatial skills
  – Language
  – Cognitive motor processing speed
  – Executive functioning
  – Motor abilities
  – Mood/emotional state
■ As with all neuropsychological evaluation, specific tests should be selected by a neuropsychologist to adequately address the referral question. Specific tests should validly assess the intended cognitive domain and be well standardized. Ideally, alternate forms of evaluation should be available to minimize practice effects in the case of repeated evaluations.
■ A neuropsychologist should interpret test results and make recommendations.
■ Administration of tests can be performed by well-trained technicians.
■ Screening techniques, such as the Mini-Mental State Examination (MMSE), are insufficient owing to insensitivity to subtle cognitive deficits, as well as other issues.

■ Patient self-report has also been found to be a poor indicator of the presence and degree of cognitive dysfunction.
■ Social presentation, such as the ability to participate in casual conversation, is also an unreliable indicator of cognitive functioning.

Treatment
■ Patient and caregiver education regarding the nature of cognitive difficulties in cancer patients is important, including education regarding the potential safety risks associated with cognitive impairment.
■ Cognitive rehabilitation techniques focusing on compensating for cognitive impairment are typically utilized, and these techniques have largely been adapted from those used in traumatic brain injury and stroke populations. However, because the cognitive impairment seen in brain tumor patients is often less severe and more variable than that seen in traumatic brain injury and stroke patients, care should be taken to target such techniques to the individual patient. Traumatic brain injury and stroke neurorehabilitation programs are often not appropriate for the needs of brain tumor patients.
■ Stimulant medications have been used to decrease fatigue, and may increase motor activity, but studies have suggested that cognition may not be enhanced.
■ Addressing obstacles which may further exacerbate cognitive impairment, including psychological factors, fatigue, sleep disorders, pain, and medication effects, is important.

Prognosis
■ The great majority of patients with chemotherapy-related mild cognitive dysfunction will have returned to baseline in approximately 1 year following completion of chemotherapy. However, there is evidence that a minority of patients will experience persistent cognitive difficulties at least 10 years later. To date, the relationship between chemotherapy-related mild cognitive dysfunction and the development of dementia later in life is unclear.
■ Unlike other neurological populations, such as traumatic brain injury (TBI) and cerebrovascular accident (CVA) patients, few studies have been conducted regarding recovery of cognitive deficits in the brain tumor population. Prognosis for cognitive deficits related to brain tumors or neurooncological etiologies will be highly variable and depend on the

severity of presenting cognitive symptoms, disease progression, and many other individual factors. Despite this variability, cognitive functioning has been found to have prognostic significance in brain tumor patients. For instance, in a recent study of older glioblastoma multiforme (GBM) patients, those with preoperative cognitive deficits had an 80% decreased survival rate compared with patients without cognitive deficits. In addition, studies have found that cognitive decline precedes radiographic progression.

■ The prognosis for recovery of cognitive deficits related to the late delayed effects of cranial radiation, that is, cognitive deficits presenting 1 to 2 years following radiotherapy, is poor. These deficits are more likely to be irreversible, and are sometimes progressive.

Helpful Hints

■ Cognitive dysfunction is common in cancer patients. Neuropsychological testing should be considered any time a patient, family member, or treatment team raise concerns for cognitive difficulties.

■ Cognitive functioning is often the most relevant issue for ability to return to work, return to school, return to driving, and ability to live independently. Neuropsychological testing can be used to make important functional recommendations for patients and their families to improve their quality of life, evaluate capacity to make medical decisions, assist in discharge planning (safety and supervision recommendations), disability evaluations, and evaluate whether poor compliance is related to cognitive factors.

■ Cognitive functioning is also an important factor in quality of life—even mild cognitive deficits can significantly impact quality of life and lead to a loss of independence. In addition, patients who sustain cognitive changes often experience a distressing change in sense of self.

■ Neuropsychological evaluation offers an objective method of measuring cognition utilizing well-validated instruments which can account for age, education, premorbid IQ, primary language or cultural differences, aphasic symptoms, and so forth. Screening tests are insensitive to subtle cognitive changes, and patient self-report as well as social presentation are often unreliable indicators of cognitive functioning. Neuroimaging results also offer no information regarding cognition and level of functioning.

■ Neuropsychological data can be used to monitor cognitive recovery, as well as the usefulness of cognitive rehabilitation techniques.

Suggested Reading

Meyers CA, Perry JR, eds. *Cognition and Cancer*. New York, NY: Cambridge University Press; 2008.

III: Cancer- or Treatment-Related Symptoms

Cranial Nerve XI Injury Associated With Radical Neck Dissection

Ying Guo MD MS

Description

Patients having radical neck dissection (RND) undergo resection of the spinal accessory nerve with resulting denervation of the trapezius muscle and destabilization of the scapula. Modified radical neck dissection (MRND) and selective neck dissection (SND) were designed to avoid spinal accessory nerve injury; however, even with this approach injury to the spinal accessory nerve can still occur.

Etiology/Types

- Partial or complete accessory nerve damage (subfascial branches of the cervical plexus severed as part of RND).

Epidemiology

- Of those patients who underwent RND:
  - 31% experienced severe limitations of shoulder mobility and pain.
  - 41% suffered only mild discomfort.
  - 28% were free of complaints.

Pathogenesis

- Loss of trapezius muscle function causes the scapulae to move laterally, that is, lateral scapular winging.

Clinical Features

Patients can present with shoulder pain and discomfort, weakness, decreased range of motion, and decreased ability to perform overhead activities.

Diagnosis

- Trapezius muscle weakness
- Drooping shoulder at rest
- Unable to abduct shoulder more than 90°
- Winged scapula (lateral displacement, more in the upper portion of the scapula), more prominent when abducting the shoulder (Figure 24.1).
- Inability to perform overhead activity

Differential diagnosis

- Medial winging: due to long thoracic nerve injury, causing serratus anterior weakness. With shoulder flexed, the patient pushes against a wall, the entire scapula will move medially and superiorly (Figure 24.2).

- Lateral winging: due to dorsal scapular nerve injury, causing rhomboid weakness. When the shoulder is moved from full flexion to extension, the scapula moves laterally, especially the inferior angle (Figure 24.3).

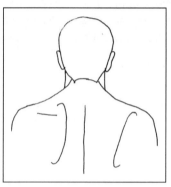

Figure 24.1   Lateral scapular winging from trapezius weakness.

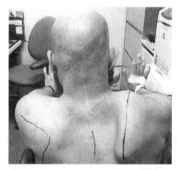

Figure 24.2   Medial scapular winging from serratus weakness.

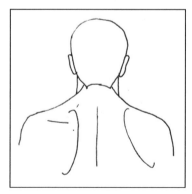

Figure 24.3   Lateral scapular winging from rhomboid weakness.

History
- RND, sometimes after MRND, SND
- Pain and lack of shoulder abduction interfere with activities of daily living.

Examination
- When sitting or standing with the patient's arms resting next to their body, an asymmetrical neckline with drooping of the affected shoulder can be noticed.
- Patient has difficulty abducting shoulder. Active shoulder abduction is limited in the majority of patients to 80° to 90°.
- Arm abduction and external rotation against resistance causes the scapula to move laterally with the superior angle more laterally than the inferior angle.
- Electromyographic testing of the trapezius muscle typically shows resting denervation potentials in complete injury to CN XI. Can also show decreased motor unit recruitment and polyphasic motor unit potentials during volitional activity in the chronic phase.

Treatment
- Conservative treatments: not very effective
  - Physical therapy: avoid activation of pectoralis; strengthening of the levator scapulae and rhomboids
  - Transcutaneous nerve stimulation
  - External support such as a shoulder orthosis
  - Medication for pain control: nonsteroidal anti-inflammatory drugs (NSAIDs) and opioids
- Surgical exploration and nerve repair
- Scapulothoracic fusion

Prognosis
- Fair

Helpful Hints
- Inform patient of the possibility of nerve damage prior to surgery.
- Maintain range of motion of the shoulder.
- Use electromyography to help predict prognosis.

Suggested Readings
Erisen L, Basel B, Irdesel J, et al. Shoulder function after accessory nerve-sparing neck dissections. *Head Neck.* 2004;26(11):967.

Kizilay A, Kalcioglu MT, Saydem L, Ersoy Y. A new shoulder orthosis for paralysis of the trapezius muscle after radical neck dissection: A preliminary report. *Eur Arch Otorrhinolaryngol.* 2006;263:477–480.

Krause HR. Shoulder-arm-syndrome after radical neck dissection: Its relation with the innervation of the trapezius muscle. *Int J Oral Maxillofac Surg.* 1992;21(5):276.

III: Cancer- or Treatment-Related Symptoms

Dyspnea

David Hui MD MSc FRCPC

Description

Dyspnea is a subjective awareness of difficulty breathing, which may be associated with the distressing sensation of suffocation.

Epidemiology

- Dyspnea is present in 20% to 50% of patients at the time of diagnosis of advanced cancer, and in 50% to 70% of cancer patients in the last 6 weeks of life.

Pathogenesis

- The following mechanisms can increase the sensation of dyspnea in the somatosensory cortex
  - Activation of chemoreceptors (low P_aO_2, high P_aCO_2) in the carotid and aortic bodies and centrally
  - Activation of mechanoceptors, irritant receptors, juxtacapillary receptors, and baroreceptors lining the airways, lung, and pulmonary arteries
  - Activation of chest wall receptors
  - Neuroventilatory dissociation (i.e., drive to breath greater than ability to breath)
  - Activation of amygdala (e.g., anxiety)

Risk Factors

- Lung cancer
- Mesothelioma
- Comorbidities (e.g., chronic obstructive pulmonary disease [COPD])

Clinical Features

- Dyspnea is associated with fatigue, anxiety, depression, and delirium.
- Limited mobility
- Inability to work
- Interrupted speech
- Decreased quality of life

Diagnosis

Differential diagnosis

- Respiratory:
  - Airway—airway obstruction, acute bronchitis, COPD, asthma
  - Parenchyma—pneumonia, lymphangitic carcinomatosis, acute respiratory distress syndrome, interstitial pneumonitis
  - Vascular—pulmonary embolism, pulmonary hypertension, superior vena cava syndrome
  - Pleural—pleural effusion, pneumothorax
- Cardiac:
  - Pericardial—pericardial effusion, tamponade
  - Myocardial—heart failure exacerbation, myocardial infarction
  - Valvular—aortic stenosis
- Abdominal—ascites
- Neuromuscular—cachexia
- Systemic—sepsis, metabolic acidosis, anemia
- Psychogenic—anxiety

History

- Persistent dyspnea: intensity (e.g., numeric rating scale from 0–10, in which 0 = no dyspnea and 10 = worst possible), onset, quality (e.g., chest tightness, increased work of breathing, air hunger, suffocation)
- Episodic dyspnea: intensity, number of episodes per day, duration per episode, triggers (activity, anxiety)
- Previous and current treatments: opioids, oxygen, bronchodilators, steroids, other nonpharmacologic treatments
- Impact: level of function (e.g., walking distance), avoidance of activities
- Comorbidities and smoking history

Examination

- Important note: physiologic changes are only weakly associated with patients' subjective sensation of dyspnea.
- Vital signs (heart rate, respiratory rate, blood pressure, oxygen saturation, oxygen level)
- Cachexia, accessory muscle use, paradoxical breathing, nasal flaring, grunting, look of fear
- Respiratory examination
- Cardiac examination

Testing

- Directed based on differential diagnosis, history, and physical examination
- Chest x-ray
- CT chest
- Echocardiogram: if pericardial effusion suspected

Treatment

- Underlying causes:
  - Antineoplastic therapy for cancer
  - Anticoagulation for pulmonary embolism
  - Antibiotics for pneumonia
  - Endoscopic interventions for central airway obstruction
- Symptomatic treatments:
  - Opioids: strong evidence to support that systemic (but not nebulized) opioids can decrease the sensation of shortness of breath. Opioids should be considered as first-line treatment. The doses and titration schedules for opioids are similar to those used for pain management.
  - Supplemental oxygen: useful to decrease dyspnea in hypoxemic patients only. High-flow oxygen and noninvasive ventilation represent novel oxygen delivery options.
  - Corticosteroids: may be useful although the evidence supporting the use of corticosteroids remains limited.
  - Bronchodilators: for patients with bronchoconstriction
  - Others: pulmonary rehabilitation (e.g., breathing exercises, inspiratory muscle training, postural drainage, energy conservation, patient education and support), nursing interventions, handheld fan
  - Palliative sedation: for patients with severe refractory dyspnea despite a trial of all other reasonable therapeutic options. Palliative sedation should only be given after detailed discussions with the patient/family members and health care team.

Prognosis

- Dyspnea is an important prognostic factor in patients with advanced cancer.
- Patients who have dyspnea at rest have a shorter survival compare to those who only have dyspnea on exertion, who in turn have a shorter survival compared to patients without dyspnea.

Helpful Hints

- Dyspnea is one of the most common and distressing symptoms in patients with advanced cancer.
- Dyspnea is often multifactorial in nature. Patients do not have to be hypoxemic to have dyspnea. Cachexia is often an overlooked contributor.
- Distinction should be made between persistent and episodic dyspnea; 20% of patients have persistent dyspnea only, 60% have episodic dyspnea only, and the remaining 20% have both.
- Routine screening and early management with a multidisciplinary team (supportive/palliative care, pulmonary medicine, medical/radiation oncology, physiotherapy/occupational therapy) are recommended.
- Respiratory depression is unlikely with opioids except with rapid titration. Naloxone should be given if patients have low respiratory rate (less than 6/minute), constricted pupils, and decreased level of consciousness.

Suggested Readings

Ben-Aharon I, Gafter-Gvili A, Paul M, et al. Interventions for alleviating cancer-related dyspnea: A systematic review. *J Clin Oncol.* 2008;26(14):2396–2404.

Del Fabbro E, Dalal S, Bruera E. Symptom control in palliative care—Part III: Dyspnea and delirium. *J Palliat Med.* 2006;9(2):422–436.

Mahler DA, Selecky PA, Harrod CG, et al. American College of Chest Physicians consensus statement on the management of dyspnea in patients with advanced lung or heart disease. *Chest.* 2010;137(3):674–691.

Parshall MB, Schwartzstein RM, Adams L, et al. An official American Thoracic Society Statement: Update on the mechanisms, assessment, and management of dyspnea. *Am J Respir Crit Care Med.* 2012;185(4):435–452.

Viola R, Kiteley C, Lloyd NS, et al. The management of dyspnea in cancer patients: A systematic review. *Support Care Cancer.* 2008;16(4):329–337.

III: Cancer- or Treatment-Related Symptoms

Emergency Medical Issues

Samir M. Haq MD ■ Ahmed Elsayem MD

Description

Emergencies in cancer patients present challenges not only diagnostically but also therapeutically. The outcome of some of these conditions is time sensitive and requires immediate attention. Practitioners caring for cancer patients must be well versed in these emergencies, as immediate treatment of them is often needed.

Presenting Signs and Symptoms

Chest pain

■ Etiology: The cancer patient may have chronic chest pain from tumor metastasis to ribs or pleura or as side effects to therapy, such as post thoracotomy pain or radiation or chemotherapy esophagitis. However, more serious medical conditions, such as myocardial infarction (MI), should not be overlooked. Other medical conditions include:
  – Cardiac: myocardial infarction (MI), aortic dissection, pericarditis
  – Pulmonary: pulmonary embolism (PE), pneumothorax, pleuritis
  – Gastrointestinal: gastroesophageal reflux disease, esophageal spasm/rupture, biliary colic
  – Other: costochondritis, anxiety, herpes zoster
■ Workup: electrocardiogram (EKG), cardiac enzymes, complete blood count (CBC), possible chest CT, possible echocardiogram
■ Emergency considerations: If known cardiac history or risk factors for MI, and no contraindications, aspirin and nitroglycerin sublingual recommended.

Dyspnea

■ Etiology: The cancer patient may have chronic shortness of breath owing to primary or metastatic lung disease, cancer therapy (e.g., radiation pneumonitis), or deconditioning. Acute worsening of dyspnea is an emergency and the following differential should be considered:
  – Pulmonary: PE, pleural effusion, chronic obstructive pulmonary disease, pneumonia, pneumothorax, asthma, airway obstruction
  – Cardiology: myocardial infarction, heart failure, pericardial effusion/tamponade, arrhythmia
  – Other: anemia, deconditioning, superior vena cava syndrome

■ Workup: pulse oximetry, chest x-ray, electrocardiogram, cardiac enzymes, possible chest CT, possible echocardiogram
■ Emergency considerations: pretest probability for PE is significantly higher in the cancer patient as compared to the general population. Have a lower threshold for chest CT with PE protocol.

Altered mental status

■ Etiology: Advanced cancer, particularly in the elderly, is one of the main causes of acute confusional state (delirium). Main causes include medications, such as opioids, benzodiazepines, or infections. Other causes of altered mental status (AMS):
  – Neurologic: stroke, seizure, new brain metastasis
  – Infectious: pneumonia, urinary tract infection (UTI), meningitis.
  – Metabolic: hepatic encephalopathy, hypercalcemia, hypoglycemia, hypernatremia
  – Other: medications, hypoxia, constipation, lack of eye glasses, hearing aids.
■ Workup: finger stick blood glucose measurement, brain CT or MRI, CBC, urinalysis, electrolytes, possible lumbar puncture
■ Emergency considerations: Assure safety of the patient and the medical staff. Stop possible contributing medications, and consider the use of antipsychotic medications, such as haloperidol, in agitated patients. Be sure to immediately check blood glucose levels as this can be readily treated. Consider UTI, constipation, or simple items such as the absence of eye glasses or hearing aids in elderly patients

Fever and hypotension

■ Etiology: Cancer patients, especially those who have received recent chemotherapy, are at greater risk of infections. Pneumonia is the most common infection. Patients with hematologic cancer, such as leukemia or lymphoma are frequently neutropenic, with an absolute neutrophil count less than 500/mcL. Fever could be an early sign of severe infection and can become fatal if not treated immediately. Severe infection can lead to hypotension and shock.
  – Infectious: pneumonia, UTI, indwelling line or port infection, cellulitis, occult abscess

– Other: directly from malignancy (tumor fever), medications, blood transfusion, pulmonary embolism, neuroleptic malignant syndrome
■ Workup: CBC; blood/urine/sputum/indwelling intravenous line cultures; chest x-ray; careful physical exam, including examination of oral cavity, perirectal area, and sites of intravenous access
■ Emergency considerations: infection until proven otherwise. Typical signs of infection may not be present in neutropenic patients. Start broad spectrum antibiotics immediately in neutropenic patients.

Bleeding
■ Etiology: Generally, cancer patients are at increased risk of bleeding. Thrombocytopenia is frequent in patients with hematologic malignancies or after recent chemotherapy. Massive bleeding is rare but sometimes can occur from the upper or lower gastrointestinal tract or the lungs. In head and neck cancer patients, severe hemorrhage can result from tumors eroding through major vessels.
– Hematologic: thrombocytopenia from chemotherapy or malignant invasion of bone marrow; coagulopathy from disseminated intravascular coagulation, liver dysfunction, anticoagulant medication
– Other: direct tumor invasion into blood vessels or airway
■ Workup: Quantify the amount of blood lost. CBC, type and cross match, prothrombin and partial thromboplastin time, liver function tests
■ Emergency considerations: Obtain good IV access with large-bore needles and start IV fluids; protect airway with intubation for massive hemoptysis.

Cancer-Specific Emergencies

Metastatic spinal cord compression
■ Etiology: compression of spinal cord or cauda equina by metastatic tumors; the most common implicated cancers are breast, lung, prostate, and multiple myeloma
■ Clinical findings: back pain (often worse with recumbence), weakness, sensory changes, and change in bowel or bladder function
■ Diagnosis: MRI is the imaging modality of choice, and imaging of the entire spine is preferable. A CT myelogram can be used if MRI is not readily available.
■ Treatment: Immediate treatment is required to preserve neurologic function. Start dexamethasone 10 mg IV followed by 4 mg every 6 hours. Immediate consultation of neurosurgery and/or radiation therapy is needed.

Tumor lysis syndrome
■ Etiology: spontaneous or more commonly treatment-induced cell death with resultant release of intracellular material. Frequently occurs during treatment of leukemia, lymphoma, or bulky solid tumors.
■ Diagnosis: based on laboratory findings of hyperkalemia, hyperphosphatemia, hyperuricemia, hypocalcemia, and rapid progression to renal failure
■ Treatment: aggressive hydration prior to and during chemotherapy administration. Either rasburicase or allopurinol can be used to lower uric acid levels. Frequent monitoring and correction of electrolyte abnormalities are recommended.

Hypercalcemia of malignancy
■ Etiology: local osteolysis of bone from metastatic lesions, tumor production of parathyroid hormone-related peptide, or tumor production of calcitriol (1,25-dihydroxyvitamin D). Commonly implicated cancers include breast, lung cancers, and multiple myeloma.
■ Clinical findings: Signs and symptoms are similar to other causes of hypercalcemia and include dehydration, weakness, constipation, arrhythmia, AMS, and coma.
■ Diagnosis: Serum and ionized calcium levels will be elevated. Measure intact parathyroid hormone and parathyroid hormone-related peptide.
■ Treatment: Intravenous fluid replacement is important as dehydration is common. Symptomatic hypercalcemia can be treated with calcitonin for immediate correction and bisphosphonates for longer-term treatment.

Suggested Readings
Breitbart W, Alici Y. Evidence-based treatment of deliriumin patients with cancer. *J Clin Oncol.* 2012 Apr 10;30(11):1206–1214.
Cairo MS, Coiffier B, Reiter A, et al. Recommendations for the evaluation of risk and prophylaxis of tumour lysis syndrome (TLS) in adults and children with malignant diseases: An expert TLS panel consensus. *Br J Haematol.* 2010 May;149(4):578–586.
Cervantes A, Chirivella I. Oncological emergencies. *Ann Oncol.* 2004;15(suppl 4):iv299–iv306.
Sipsas NV, Bodey GP, Kontoyiannis DP. Perspectives for the management of febrile neutropenic patients with cancer in the 21st century. *Cancer.* 2005 Mar 15;103(6):1103–1113.
Stewart AF. Clinical practice. Hypercalcemia associated with cancer. *N Engl J Med.* 2005 Jan 27;352(4):373–379.
Wilkinson AN, Viola R, Brundage MD. Managing skeletal related events resulting from bone metastases. *BMJ.* 2008 Nov 3;337:1101–1108.
Yahalom J, Baehring JM, Becker K, Fojo A. Oncologic emergencies. In: DeVita VT, Hellman S, Rosenberg SA, eds. *Cancer: Principles & Practice of Oncology.* 9th ed. Philadelphia, PA: Lippincott Williams & Wilkins; 2011:2123–2152.

III: Cancer- or Treatment-Related Symptoms

Fatigue

Sriram Yennu MD MS

Description

Fatigue is the most common symptom in patients with cancer with a frequency varying from 60% to 90%. It is also one of the most undertreated symptoms in cancer patients. Fatigue has a substantial adverse impact on quality of life (QOL) for both patients and caregivers.

■ The National Comprehensive Cancer Network (NCCN) defines cancer-related fatigue as a "distressing, persistent, subjective sense of physical, emotional, and/or cognitive tiredness or exhaustion related to cancer or cancer treatment that is not proportional to activity and that interferes with usual functioning."

Etiology

■ Fatigue is most often a multidimensional symptom, often with multiple causes.
■ Among these patients, correlative studies have shown an association of fatigue with pain, dyspnea, anorexia, and psychological symptoms.
■ Other major contributors may include inflammation, anemia, and medications such as anticholinergics, antihistamines, anticonvulsants, neuroleptics, opioids, central-antagonists, beta-blockers, diuretics, antidepressants, muscle relaxants, and benzodiazepines.

Assessment

■ A comprehensive history and physical examination should be undertaken to ascertain the various organ systems affected by the underlying disease, comorbid conditions, and also to direct the diagnostic workup.
■ Fatigue severity can be quantified by using the 0 to 10 visual analog scale.
■ Use of simple tools such as the Edmonton Symptom Assessment Scale may be helpful for a more comprehensive assessment of fatigue in both clinical and research settings (see Table 27.1).

Diagnosis

Differential diagnosis

■ Potentially reversible medical conditions such as anemia, infection, pain, anorexia, insomnia, and psychological symptoms should be identified and appropriately treated.

Treatment

■ If a cause is not reversible or apparent, symptomatic treatment is appropriate.
■ The treatment of fatigue should ideally involve an interdisciplinary team approach with active participation by the clinician, nurse, psychiatric counselor, social worker, chaplain, physical therapist, and occupational therapist.

Treatment of anemia

■ Optimal management of symptomatic anemia requires an accurate diagnosis to identify potentially remediable causes (e.g., ongoing blood loss, hemolysis, or deficiency of iron, folic acid, or vitamin B_{12}).
■ If a potentially treatable cause cannot be identified, treatment options include red blood cell (RBC) transfusion, or for selected patients, an erythropoiesis stimulating agent (ESA).
■ *Transfusions* of packed RBCs can improve fatigue that is due to anemia, at least in the short term.
■ Treatment with ESAs can be beneficial in relieving fatigue and improving QOL in patients with chronic anemia that is related to cancer chemotherapy. ESAs are significantly associated with improvement of fatigue, with maximum benefit occurring when the hemoglobin is improved to 12 g/dL.
  – Use of these agents has become controversial in certain patients with cancer, in particular those with anemia unrelated to chemotherapy and in those receiving myelosuppressive chemotherapy with the intent of cure because of concerns about thromboembolic side effects, higher mortality rates, and the possibility of adverse cancer outcomes.

Symptomatic treatment

■ Pharmacologic approaches:
  – There are a limited number of pharmacologic agents that have demonstrated efficacy in the treatment of fatigue in cancer patients.
  – The lack of good studies is related to the complex nature of fatigue in this population, and paucity of research on cancer-related fatigue.

Table 27.1 Edmonton Symptom Assessment System—Revised

Please circle the number that best describes how you feel NOW:

No Pain	0	1	2	3	4	5	6	7	8	9	10	Worst Possible Pain
No Tiredness (*Tiredness = lack of energy*)	0	1	2	3	4	5	6	7	8	9	10	Worst Possible Tiredness
No Drowsiness (*Drowsiness = feeling sleepy*)	0	1	2	3	4	5	6	7	8	9	10	Worst Possible Drowsiness
No Nausea	0	1	2	3	4	5	6	7	8	9	10	Worst Possible Nausea
No Lack of Appetite	0	1	2	3	4	5	6	7	8	9	10	Worst Possible Lack of Appetite
No Shortness of Breath	0	1	2	3	4	5	6	7	8	9	10	Worst Possible Shortness of Breath
No Depression (*Depression = feeling sad*)	0	1	2	3	4	5	6	7	8	9	10	Worst Possible Depression
No Anxiety (*Anxiety = feeling nervous*)	0	1	2	3	4	5	6	7	8	9	10	Worst Possible Anxiety
Best Well-Being (*Well-being = how you feel overall*)	0	1	2	3	4	5	6	7	8	9	10	Worst Possible Well-Being
No _____ Other Problem (*for example, constipation*)	0	1	2	3	4	5	6	7	8	9	10	Worst Possible _____

Source: Reprinted from Watanabe S. A multicenter study comparing two numerical versions of the Edmonton Symptom Assessments System in Palliative Care Patients. *J Pain Symptom Manage*, 2011;41(2):456–468. Reprinted with permission from Elsevier.

- Glucocorticoids:
  - Preliminary studies have found that glucocorticoids reduce symptoms such as fatigue, pain, and nausea, and improve appetite and overall QOL in patients with advanced cancer.
  - In a recent randomized placebo-controlled trial of 84 evaluable patients with advanced cancer, oral dexamethasone (8 mg per day for 14 days) significantly improved fatigue. Unfortunately, side effects limit the long-term use of glucocorticoids. The severity of most toxicities is dose dependent. Side effects observed in some patients include infection, oral thrush, insomnia, mood swings, myalgia, and elevation of blood glucose.
- Psychostimulants:
  - Both fatigue and depression can be treated with psychostimulants such as dextroamphetamine, methylphenidate, or modafinil.
  - Psychostimulants act rapidly, and are generally well tolerated and safe.
  - All of the available evidence shows that methylphenidate and modafinil have shown beneficial effects in patients with severe fatigue; benefit is less certain in patients with mild to moderate fatigue.
  - Methylphenidate is usually administered twice a day, at breakfast and lunch, in order to minimize nighttime insomnia (starting dose 5 mg twice a day).
  - Modafinil is typically administered as a single daily dose of 200 mg in the morning.
- Complementary medicines: Preliminary studies have suggested efficacy for American ginseng and guarana for the treatment of cancer-related fatigue. However, further long-term safety studies are needed, particularly regarding the potential for drug interactions with ginseng.

- Nonpharmacologic approaches:
  - Exercise:
    - Physical activity is important to maintain a sense of well-being and to enhance QOL.
    - Exercise (aerobic or endurance for at least 150 minutes/week) during or after curative or life-prolonging treatment was found to be effective in improving cancer-related fatigue.
  - Behavioral and psychosocial interventions:
    - Various randomized clinical trials have shown that supportive interventions (group and individual), such as education and stress management groups, coping strategies training, and behavioral interventions have been helpful for cancer patients with managing their fatigue.
- Multimodal interventions for refractory fatigue:
  - In patients with refractory fatigue, patients are likely to benefit from a combination of pharmacologic and nonpharmacologic interventions. Cognitive behavioral therapy, increased physical activity, and pharmacologic therapy aimed at countering inflammation and targeting changes in body composition should be individualized.

Helpful Hints

- Fatigue is typically a multidimensional symptom.
- If a specific cause cannot be identified, a combined pharmacological (e.g., trial of dexamethasone or methylphenidate) and nonpharmacological approach (such as exercise, cognitive behavioral therapy) is suggested.

Suggested Readings

Berger AM, Abernethy AP, Atkinson A, et al. Cancer-related fatigue. *J Natl Compr Canc Netw.* 2010;8:904–931.

Bruera E, Yennurajalingam S. Challenge of managing cancer-related fatigue. *J Clin Oncol.* 2010;28:3671–3672.

Febrile Neutropenia in Acute Leukemia Patients

Khanh D. Vu MD

Description

Neutropenia is defined as an absolute neutrophil count (ANC) of less than 500 neutrophils/mL or ANC of 1,000/mL or less, but rapidly decreasing. *Febrile neutropenia* or *neutropenic fever* is defined as neutropenia with:

- A single temperature higher than 38.3°C
- A temperature of more than 38°C persistent for more than 1 hour
- Three or more temperatures higher than 38°C within a 24-hour period, taken at least 4 hours apart

- Hematologic malignancy and stem cell transplant patients are considered high-risk categories.

Etiology

- Neutropenia can be disease and/or treatment related.
- The occurrence, degree of, and duration of neutropenia are dependent on the myelosuppressive nature of the chemotherapeutic agents. Treatment of acute leukemia routinely requires intensive, cytotoxic chemotherapy and hence, neutropenia occurs in the majority of acute leukemia patients.

Epidemiology

- In febrile neutropenia, an infectious source is identified in only 30% of the episodes. It is believed that approximately 80% of the identified infections arise from the patient's endogenous flora.

Pathogenesis

- Febrile neutropenia occurs because of host defense impairments. This includes:
  - Disease-related neutrophil dysfunction
  - Altered cellular and humoral immunity
  - Treatment-related neutropenia
  - Altered mucosa (predominantly gastrointestinal tract)
  - Altered skin integrity
  - Anemia
  - Thrombocytopenia (poor wound healing)

Risk Factors (for Febrile Neutropenia)

- Age of 60 years or older
- Relapsed or refractory leukemia
- Cytotoxic chemotherapy
- High-dose corticosteroids
- Splenectomy
- Indwelling central venous catheter (CVC)
- Empiric use of antibiotic prophylaxis, particularly quinolone based
- Transfusions of blood products

Clinical Features

- Sites that are often the foci of infection are the oropharynx, gastrointestinal tract, paranasal sinuses, lungs, urinary tract, and skin (particularly perineum, perirectal, and vascular catheter insertion site). Signs and symptoms are usually associated with these sites. Because neutropenia alters the host's inflammatory response, signs and symptoms of infections can initially be very subtle or missing.
- Shaking rigors may precede fever and may continue to occur with fever.
- Fever may not occur in patients on corticosteroids or in the elderly.
- Elderly patients may present with somnolence and confusion.

Diagnosis

History

- Document factors associated with increased risk of infection include age greater than 65, type and stage of malignancy, chemotherapy regimen, and comorbid organ dysfunction.

Physical

- Localizing signs and symptoms of infection, vital signs, signs of impending sepsis.

Testing

- Complete blood count (CBC), platelet, and differential [ANC = (total white blood cells [WBC]) × (% neutrophils)].

- Blood cultures—if patient has CVC, simultaneous blood cultures should be obtained from the catheter as well as peripheral site.
- Culture from other appropriate sites as per clinical correlation (e.g., sputum, nasal washings, urine, stool for *Clostridium difficile*)
- Cytomegalovirus (CMV) antigen detection or molecular amplification assay if clinically indicated
- Chest x-ray
- Other imaging, such as CT sinuses, CT chest, or CT abdomen and pelvis as indicated
- Skin biopsy or bronchoscopy should be performed as clinically indicated

Treatment

- Treatment of febrile neutropenia in leukemia patients should be discussed with and/or addressed by the leukemia specialist, leukemia hospitalist, and/or infectious diseases consultant.
- Initial treatment with monotherapy (e.g., third or fourth generation cephalosporin or carbapenem) would be appropriate in stable patients.
- Combination therapy (third- or fourth-generation cephalosporin or carbapenem plus an aminoglycoside or fluoroquinolone) seems to be more effective in patients with clinical signs suggestive of gram-negative sepsis.
- Gram-positive coverage (e.g., vancomycin, daptomycin, or linezolid) should be added in the presence of signs of catheter-related infections, mucositis, other skin or soft tissue infections, suspected gram-positive pneumonia, known colonization of penicillin-resistant pneumococci or methicillin-resistant staphylococci, hemodynamic instability, or signs of sepsis.
- Antivirals and antifungals are often continued as prophylaxis or escalated empirically. Documented viral and fungal infections should be treated with disease-specific antivirals and antifungals, respectively.
- The use of growth factors (G-CSF or GM-CSF) and/or WBC transfusions should be considered at the discretion of the leukemia specialist, leukemia hospitalist, or infectious diseases consultant.

Prognosis

- The risk of developing complications correlates with the degree of neutropenia and the duration of neutropenia (the lower the ANC and the longer the duration of neutropenia, the higher the risk of complications). Other variables which may increase morbidity and mortality include older age, serious independent comorbidities, and/or uncontrolled relapsed and refractory leukemia.

Helpful Hints

- Patients do not need to be placed in reverse isolation. However, hand hygiene and standard barrier precautions should be followed. Plants and flowers (fresh or dried) should not be allowed in the rooms. Limit exposure to family or health care workers who have signs and symptoms of a potentially contagious illness.
- After intensive chemotherapy, the neutrophil nadir and recovery is variable for different chemotherapeutic agents. Often, the neutrophil count will nadir around day 14. Recovery of the ANC of more than 1,000 may occur by day 21 in patients with acute lymphocytic leukemia but often later for patients with acute myelogenous leukemia. Patients with relapsed and refractory leukemia frequently have persistent neutropenia.
- Infections (e.g., skin infections and pneumonias) may temporarily worsen as the neutrophil count recovers.
- CMV infection occurs more frequently in chronic leukemias but may also occur in acute leukemias. Patients may be asymptomatic except for fever or may present with an array of *itis*es, such as retinitis, hepatitis, encephalitis. Consider this in patients after stem cell transplant or in a leukemia patient with an unexpected decrease in platelet count.
- Suspect invasive fungal infections in leukemia patients, particularly acute myelogenous leukemia, who remain febrile despite 4 to 7 days of broad spectrum antibiotics.
- Daptomycin is not effective for pulmonary infections. It can also be associated with myopathy; therefore, monitor creatine phosphokinase and use with caution in patients receiving other drugs that are associated with myopathy (e.g., statins).

Suggested Readings

Feifield AG, Bow EJ, Sepkowitz KA, et al. Clinical practice guideline for the use of antimicrobial agents in neutropenic patients with cancer: 2010 update by the Infectious Diseases Society of America. *Clin Infec Dis.* 2011;52:e56–e93.

O'Brien S, Thomas DA, Ravandi F, et al. Results of hyperfractionated cyclophosphamide, vincristine, doxorubicin, and dexamethasone regimen in elderly patients with acute lymphocytic leukemia. *Cancer.* 2008;113(8):2097–2101.

Free Tissue Transfer

Edward I. Chang MD ▪ Julie A. Moeller PT DPT ▪ David W. Chang MD

Description

Following free tissue transfer, rehabilitation is a critical component in the recovery of patients to restore mobility and performance of activities of daily living. The precise therapeutic regimen is dependent on the donor site as well as the recipient site.

Donor-Site Precautions

TRAM (transverse rectus abdominis myocutaneous) or DIEP (deep inferior epigastric perforators) abdominal donor site

▪ Avoid heavy lifting and/or strenuous activity for minimum of 6 weeks, abdominal precautions for up to 6 weeks to minimize chance of developing hernia or a bulge.
▪ Maintain some flexion at the hips to avoid tension on skin closure until cleared by surgeon.

Free fibula osteocutaneous flap donor site

▪ Nonweight bearing on donor leg until cleared by surgeon if donor site skin grafted.
▪ Keep leg elevated at all times for 5 to 7 days, especially if donor site skin grafted.
▪ Dangling protocol with limited duration of leg placed in dependent position—to be advanced under guidance of plastic surgeon and therapist.

Anterolateral thigh or gracilis donor site

▪ No restrictions in weight-bearing status or ambulation.

Free forearm donor site

▪ Keep arm elevated at all times.
▪ Splint arm in neutral position (wrist extension, metacarpophalangeal flexion and interphalangeal extension or fingers free) for 1 to 2 weeks until skin graft has healed.
▪ Nonweight bearing use of arm until skin graft has healed, 1 to 2 weeks.

Recipient-Site Precautions

Breast recipient site

▪ Support bra without an underwire for 2 to 4 weeks following operation
▪ Partial weight bearing of upper extremity on the side of the reconstructed breast until cleared by surgeon

Head and neck recipient site

▪ Head of bed elevation to 30°
▪ Limit turning of head, or flexion and extension. Keep head midline.
▪ No ties, tubes, nasal cannulas around neck.

Extremity recipient site

▪ Keep reconstructed leg elevated at all times.
▪ No tight dressings, splints, or braces around proximal extremity that can act as a tourniquet compromising perfusion of the flap.
▪ Placement of splint or brace to be coordinated with plastic surgeon and therapist to immobilize extremity without compression.
▪ Nonweight-bearing use of reconstructed extremity and dangling protocol to be determined under guidance of the plastic surgeon and therapist.
▪ Dangling protocol to be determined under guidance of plastic surgeon and therapist.

Helpful Hints

▪ Heavy exertion and exercise can increase blood pressure and lead to bleeding and hematoma which can compromise flap perfusion and may place breast reconstruction patients at risk for developing a hernia or a bulge.
▪ Placing extremity in dependent position too soon will cause swelling that can lead to flap congestion or poor skin graft healing owing to edema.
▪ In head and neck patients after receiving free flap, extreme range of motion of the neck can increase chance of dehiscence, kinking, or avulsion of the anastomosis.

III: Cancer- or Treatment-Related Symptoms

Gastrointestinal: Constipation

Carolina Gutierrez MD

Definition
Infrequent and difficult passage of hard stool
- Fewer than three stools/week
- Hard stool
- Straining/difficulty with evacuation
- Feeling of incomplete evacuation
- Unproductive urges
- Infrequency of urges

Etiology/Types
- Structural: obstruction, pelvic mass, radiation fibrosis, anorectal pain
- Medication related: Opioid side effect, anticholinergics, chemotherapy (vinca alkaloids), others
- Metabolic: diabetes, hypothyroidism, dehydration, hypercalcemia, hypokalemia
- Neurologic: brain tumors, spinal cord involvement, cauda equina syndrome, peripheral nervous system involvement
- Related to progression of disease: changes in mental status, decreased patient mobility, metastasis (obstruction, compression), decreased gastrointestinal motility
- Intake related: changes in diet, decreased fiber, dehydration
- Weakness, inactivity
- Confusion, depression
- Unfamiliar toilet arrangement, access and ability to get to the toilet

Epidemiology
- General population:
  - Affects 40% of patients referred to palliative care
  - Affects 90% of patients treated with opioids
  - Prevalence of constipation 2% to 27% in North America
  - More common in older patients and women

Pathophysiology
- Normal bowel movements involve coordination of:
  - Motility: circular and longitudinal contractions:
    - Central nervous system
    - Peripheral nervous system:
      - Sympathetic: storage
      - Parasympathetic: colonic motility
    - Somatic innervation
    - Intrinsic enteric nervous system
    - Meissner's plexus: submucosal
    - Auerbach's plexus: intramuscular
    - Mucosal transit: prolonged bowel transit can result in desiccation of bowel content.
    - Defecation reflexes

Pathogenesis
Intrinsic or extrinsic processes can deregulate motility, mucosal transit, and/or defecation reflexes.

Diagnosis
Rome III Diagnostic Criteria can be used for diagnosis
- Two or more symptoms during the last 3 months in at least 25% of defecations:
  - Straining
  - Hard stools
  - Sensation of incomplete evacuation
  - Sensation of blockage
  - Use of manual maneuvers (digital evacuation, support of the pelvic floor, etc.)
  - Fewer than three bowel movements per week

Differential diagnosis
- Obstruction
- Diverticulitis
- Irritable bowel syndrome
- Crohn's disease
- Ogilvie syndrome

History
- Knowledge of previous bowel pattern
- Bowel diary
- Abdominal distension, abdominal fullness, abdominal or back pain
- Anorexia, nausea, and/or vomiting
- Urinary retention/incontinence
- Delirium/confusion
- Overflow diarrhea

Examination
- Abdominal exam: distension, firmness, tenderness, bowel sounds
- Rectal exam: inspection and digital rectal exam (caution with neutropenia and thrombocytopenia)

Testing

- Abdominal x-ray: can show amount of stool and localization in the colon and can rule out obstruction.
- Metabolic panel, including calcium
- Colonoscopy to rule out malignancy and/or disimpact

Treatment

- Education:
  - Toilet training
  - Biofeedback
- Correction of medical problems, including metabolic abnormalities
- Adequate hydration
- Modification of environmental factors
  - Access to bathroom
  - Bedside commode
- Diet modifications:
  - Fiber (can increase bloating)
  - Increase oral intake, prunes, and so forth
- Medications:
  - Bulk–forming agents: methylcellulose, psyllium, polycarbophil
  - Stool softener: docusate
  - Osmotic: lactulose, polyethylene glycol, sorbitol, magnesium citrate, magnesium sulfate, sodium sulfate
  - Emollient: mineral oil

- Stimulants: anthraquinones (senna, cascara), bisacodyl
- Prokinetics: metoclopramide
- Opioid antagonist: methylnaltrexone, naloxone
- Suppository/enema (caution with neutropenia and thrombocytopenia)
- Disimpaction (caution with neutropenia and thrombocytopenia)
- Example: opioid-induced constipation
  - First step: stool softener and/or laxative
  - Second step: osmotic agent
  - Third step: suppository/enema

Helpful Hints

- When prescribing opioids always counsel patient on constipation prophylaxis
- Constipation is a subjective complaint requiring thorough evaluation.
- Constipation can present as overflow diarrhea, nausea, decreased appetite, headache, shoulder or back pain.

Suggested Readings

Mancini I, Bruera E. Constipation in advanced cancer patients. *Support Care Cancer.* 1998;6(4):356–364.

Wald A. Pathophysiology, diagnosis and current management of chronic constipation. *Nat Clin Pract Gastroenterol Hepatol.* 2006;3(2):90–100.

III: Cancer- or Treatment-Related Symptoms

Gastrointestinal: Dysphagia

Jan S. Lewin PhD BRS-S

Description
Anatomic and/or neurologic disruption in the complex interaction of biomechanical, neurophysiologic, and sensory events that prevent the preparation and transit of food and liquids from the oral cavity to the stomach during the act of eating.

- Four phases or stages:
  - Oral preparatory (voluntary; mastication, manipulation, and formation)
  - Oral (voluntary; posterior bolus propulsion to the oropharynx)
  - Pharyngeal (voluntary and involuntary; initiation or "trigger" of the swallowing reflex [primarily CN IX], airway protection, and bolus entrance into cervical esophagus)
  - Esophageal (involuntary; bolus transit to stomach)
- Oropharyngeal swallow consists of the first three stages only.

Epidemiology
- Site-specific prevalence:
  - Head and neck cancer: 40% within 3 years of cancer diagnosis
  - Brain tumors: 26% with acute dysphagia; 85% at end of life
  - Esophageal cancer: 25% after surgery
- Can be first-noted symptom of head or neck, thoracic, or brain tumor

Etiology
- Generally not a single cause; rather, multiple insults resulting from the tumor itself and treatment
- Site dependent (head and neck, neurologic, and thoracic)
- Treatment dependent (surgery, radiation, chemotherapy)
- Magnitude of severity is multifactorial and variable (cumulative treatment effects, acute vs. long-term physiologic change)
- Causes: xerostomia, mucositis, reflux, odynophagia, trismus, dysgeusia, dysosmia, lymphedema, fibrosis, neuropathy, drug interactions, systemic toxicity, anatomic alterations, and sensory and motor deficits
- Sudden (trauma) versus gradual onset (progressive process, cancer)

Risk Factors
- Site of disease (brain stem, oropharynx, hypopharynx, nasopharynx, supraglottis)
- Neuromuscular disorders (multiple sclerosis, Parkinson's disease, cerebellar disorders)
- Head and neck surgery
- Head and neck lymphedema
- Connective tissue disorders (scleroderma)
- Diabetes
- Altered mental status/cognition/consciousness
- Tracheostomy
- Irradiation (head and neck, upper aerodigestive tract, lung, brain, mediastinum)
- Recurrent laryngeal/superior laryngeal nerve damage (true vocal folds [TVF] movement, laryngeal sensation)
- Substance abuse
- Smoking
- Severe deconditioning/cachexia

Signs and Symptoms
- Sensory inability to recognize food
- Inability to control and manipulate food or saliva (drooling)
- Coughing (before, during, or after swallowing)
- Recurring pneumonia
- Malnutrition
- Dehydration
- Tube feeding dependence
- Weight loss
- Gurgly, "wet" voice quality
- Nasal regurgitation
- Choking and gagging
- Increased secretions associated with mealtime
- Patient report of swallowing problems

Swallowing Facts Versus Misconceptions
- Aspiration is a symptom, not a diagnosis (must determine underlying etiology).
- Aspiration does not always preclude oral intake.
- Extended periods of NPO (nothing per os) status should be avoided (swallowing deconditioning).
- Gastrostomy tubes are indicated for prolonged dysphagia; they allow swallowing rehabilitation.

- Airway protection is not exclusively dependent on TVF closure.
- Medialization of paralyzed TVF will not always stop aspiration.
- TVF paralysis, particularly unilateral, does not always prevent a safe swallow.
- Tracheostomy tubes limit movement of larynx and trachea but do not always increase risk for aspiration.

Diagnosis
- Critical to determine rehabilitative candidacy and treatment plan
- Should be made as early as possible in patients with pretreatment tumor-related deficits and before treatment in patients at risk for treatment-related dysfunction

History
- Review of diagnosis and treatment
- Patient and family interview

Examination
- Clinical swallow examination (oral mechanism examination, swallowing observation)
- Instrumental assessment of swallowing physiology—main types
  - Modified barium swallow (MBS) study, videofluoroscopy (most widely used to evaluate entire oropharyngeal swallow, not a standard barium swallow)
  - Fiberoptic endoscopic evaluation of swallowing (FEES), videoendoscopy (disadvantage: endoscopy obstructs oral phase of the swallow, must infer physiology)
- Clinic or bedside swallowing observation, patient-reported outcomes, or performance measures alone are not reliable indicators of swallowing competency (cannot rule out silent [insensate] aspiration).

Treatment
- Technique(s) aimed at a specific goal of remediation
- Patient considerations
  - Medical/performance status
  - Disease acuity
  - Quality of life
  - Survivorship (living with cancer) versus end-of-life (palliation)
- Types:
  - Direct

- Rehabilitation/restoration—permanent effect (strengthening exercises, biofeedback)
- Compensation—transient effect (postures/adaptations, strategies, diet modifications)
- Palliation—quality of life effect (comfort/pleasure, encourage safety, minimize risk)
  - Indirect
- Change swallowing physiology without specific patient participation
- Medical or surgical (palatal prosthesis, vocal fold medialization, esophageal dilation)

Prognosis
- Early swallowing assessment and targeted intervention based on instrumental examination are critical.
- Successful treatment and rehabilitation depend on strong, expert interdisciplinary team management.
- Long-term outcomes are influenced by site of disease, type of cancer treatment, duration of swallowing deficit, and targeted swallowing intervention and monitoring.
- Patient compliance and adherence to swallowing exercise protocols are critical to success.
- Treatment based on inaccurate swallowing diagnosis is ineffective and useless.

Suggested Readings
Davie GL, Barringer DA, Lewin JS. Rehabilitation of speech and swallowing of patients with tumors of the skull base. In: Hanna EY, ed. *Comprehensive Management of Tumors of the Skull Base.* New York, NY: Informa Healthcare/Taylor & Frances; 2009:183–187.

Francis DO, Weymuller EA, Parvathaneni U, et al. Dysphagia, stricture, and pneumonia in head and neck cancer patients: Does treatment modality matter? *Ann Otol Rhinol Laryngol.* 2010;119(6):391–397.

McCabe D, Ashford J, Wheeler-Hegland K, et al. Evidenced-based systemic review: Oropharyngeal dysphagia behavioral treatments. Part IV – Impact of dysphagia on individuals' postcancer treatments. *J Rehabil Res Dev.* 2009;46(2):205–214.

McLarty AJ, Allison J, Deschamps C, et al. Esophageal resection for cancer of the esophagus: Long-term function and quality of life. *Ann Thorac Surg.* 1997;63(6):1568–1571.

Mukand JA, Blackinton DD, Crincoli MG, et al. Incidence of neurologic deficits and rehabilitation of patients with brain tumors. *Am J Phys Med Rehabil.* 2001;80(5):346.

Pace A, Lorenzo CD, Guariglia L, et al. End of life issues in brain tumor patients. *J Neurooncol.* 2009;91(1):39–43.

Rosenthal DI, Lewin JS, Eisbruch A. Prevention and treatment of dysphagia and aspiration after chemoradiation for head and neck cancer. *J Clin Oncol.* 2006;24(17):2636–2643.

III: Cancer- or Treatment-Related Symptoms

Gastrointestinal: Nutritional and Bowel Management

Benedict Konzen MD

Description

Cancer treatment is multivaried. How well we absorb nutrients depends on cancer type, location, and focal or metastatic disease. Baseline nutrition; comorbid factors—including constipation, thyroid disease, diabetes, cardiovascular status, and anticipated oncology interventions (surgery, radiation, chemotherapy/medications); and complications—such as adhesions and fibrosis also play a role.

Etiology
- Biochemical modifications
- Psychogenic association of treatment-induced emesis and foodstuffs; altered taste due to medications and chemotherapy
- Alterations in gastrointestinal motility: opiates, steroids, radiation
- Surgical: Mandibulectomy for squamous cell carcinoma of the mouth; Ivor-Lewis esophagectomy; Roux-en-Y esophago-jejunostomy; ileostomy; colostomy leading to modification in diet, digestion, and elimination
- Radiation: leads to altered mucosal absorption, motility, adhesions with potential obstruction and neurovascular compromise

Epidemiology
- 275,000 people are diagnosed with gastrointestinal cancers annually and of these, nearly 136,000 will die.
- The American Cancer Society estimated that gastrointestinal cancers accounted for 19% of all new cancers and more than 24% of all cancer deaths in 2009.
- Colorectal cancer is the third most common cancer in American men and women, accounting for 9% of all cancer deaths in the United States.

Pathogenesis
- Opiates induce xerostomia; bind to μ receptors in the gastrointestinal tract and decrease motility. This may induce nausea with early satiety and eventually emesis.
- Limited or inadequate oral fluid intake leads to obstipation. Stool becomes desiccated and unable to pass with peristaltic movement. Loose stool flowing around the obstruction is often viewed erroneously as diarrhea.
- Poor oral nutrition results in limited fiber intake and bowel regulation. Essential foodstuffs, proteins, carbohydrates, and fats are limited.
- Radiation effect to the oropharynx and esophagus can lead to mucositis and fibrosis. The patient may have dysphagia and/or have gastroesophageal reflux.
- Both surgical intervention and radiation may lead to fibrotic adhesions between the esophagus and trachea. Stenosis or tracheoesophageal fistulas may arise with ensuing bleeding or aspiration pneumonia.
- Metastatic involvement of the spine by tumor; traumatic spinal cord injury, or anatomic alteration of the spinal cord such as with tethering by radiation-induced fibrosis.

Clinical Features
- Limited nutritional intake
- Limited oral hydration
- Alterations in homeostasis by surgery, chemotherapy, radiation, or pharmacologic therapy
- Inactivity leads to increased morbidity—such as pneumonia, venous stasis, pulmonary embolus, and constipation
- Cachexia may progress despite appetite stimulants (Megace, steroids, Remeron, Marinol)

Treatment
- Familiarity with the cancer type, organ system involvement, and amount of weight loss/ascites/third space fluid gain are critical.
- Nutrition planning is key. Knowledge of prealbumin, total protein, and albumin levels are essential. Ideal body weight and additional nutritional needs must be calculated. Caloric expenditure increases with fever, recovery from surgery, and during cellular repair and growth. Protein supplements (Benefiber), renal or diabetic-based supplements (e.g., Enlive, Glucerna) should be explored. Adequate fluid intake is essential. Tachycardia may be due to dehydration and/or anemia.
- Laboratory data must be reviewed. Elevated blood urea nitrogen (BUN) may signal bleeding as well as dehydration.

- A nutritionist should follow caloric/dietary needs and intervene where necessary.
- When anorexia or emesis is pronounced, a patient may require percutaneous endoscopic gastrostomy tube placement or total parenteral nutrition/parenteral support.
- Loss of nutrition impairs healing, circulation, and proper systemic functioning—factors affecting life maintenance.

Helpful Hints

- A good history is essential, but often overlooked.
- When in doubt, obtain an acute abdominal series. Look for impaction/and or obstruction.
- Ogilvie syndrome refers to pseudodilatation of the cecum. This may be the result of surgery, chemoradiation, or medications (e.g., pain medications or steroids). The use of propulsive agents such as lactulose should be avoided.
- If (a) the patient is not pancytopenic, (b) the platelet count is greater than 50,000, (c) the fecal load is heavy but no obstruction exists, and (d) the patient is on pain medications and has increased fecal load, then consider a higher volume enema, such as a milk and molasses enema, or SMOG enema (saline + mineral oil + glycerin).
- Maintenance bowel management—especially in patients on steroids and pain medications—may include daily Senokot-S 2 to 4 tab stwice a day by mouth; MiraLax 17 g/8 oz of fluid, followed by digital stimulation and/or placement of a Dulcolax suppository ½ hour after the evening meal. Patients should also be encouraged to drink adequate amounts of water on a daily basis.

Suggested Readings

American Cancer Society: Cancer Facts and Figures 2009. Atlanta, GA: American Cancer Society; 2009.

Avila JG. Pharmacologic treatment of constipation in cancer patients. *Cancer Control*. 2004 May–Jun;11(3 suppl):10–18.

Bouras EP, Tangalos EG. Chronic constipation in the elderly. *Gastroenterol Clin North Am*. 2009 Sep;38(3):463–480.

National Health Service Fife Area Drug and Therapeutics Committee. Guidelines for the Control of Constipation in Adult Patients with Cancer. *Cancer Control*. 2004 May–Jun;11(3 suppl):24–25.

Gout

Ying Guo MD MS

Description
Gout (monosodium urate crystal deposition disease) is characterized biochemically by extracellular fluid uric acid saturation.

Etiology
- Urate crystals deposit in tissue, which leads to inflammatory and potentially destructive consequences.

Epidemiology
- Gout prevalence has been increasing in recent years and it is currently one of the most common causes of inflammatory arthritis in most developed countries. It affects up to 4% of Americans.

Pathogenesis
- Cancer and its treatment can lead to purine and/or urate overproduction.
- Myeloproliferative disorders, lymphoma, leukemia, cytotoxic drugs, warfarin are all causes.
- Excessive dietary purine ingestion contributes as well.

Risk Factors
- Older age
- Trauma, surgery, starvation, dehydration
- Fatty foods and excessive meat intake
- Obesity
- Alcohol consumption
- Hypertension alone, diuretic use, and ingestion of drugs affecting serum urate concentrations

Clinical Features

Symptoms
- Acute, severe, debilitating pain
- Great toe (first metatarsophalangeal joint) and knee involvement most frequently seen
- Difficulty with ambulation because of acute inflammation

Diagnosis

Differential diagnosis
- Septic arthritis
- Tenosynovitis
- Cellulitis
- Stress fracture
- Pseudogout and other crystalline arthritides

History
- Severe joint pain, redness, swelling, and disability
- Sudden onset, reaches maximal severity in under 24 hours; resolves within a few days to several weeks
- Lower extremity involvement; at least 80% of initial attacks involve a single joint, most often at the base of the great toe (first metatarsophalangeal joint) or the knee.

Examination
- Inflammation; severe pain, redness, swelling, warmth
- Tophus

Testing
- Synovial fluid obtained from joints or bursas (as well as material aspirated from tophaceous deposits) may be directly examined using compensated polarized light microscopy.
- Serum uric acid is more than 7 mg/dL.

Treatment
- Nonsteroidal anti-inflammatory drugs (NSAIDS)
- Colchicine (avoid in patients with end-stage renal disease)
- Intra-articular or systemic glucocorticoids
- Continue rehabilitation with other noninvolved extremities.

Prognosis
- Good

Helpful Hints
- NSAIDS are the first line of therapy for acute gout.
- Colchicine can be used at the onset of flare-up in repeat bouts.
- Steroid injection to affected single joint can be used in acute involvement.
- Hyperuricemia may lead to urolithiasis and chronic kidney disease.

Suggested Readings

Cronstein BN, Terkeltaub R. The inflammatory process of gout and its treatment. *Arthritis Res Ther.* 2006;8(suppl 1):S3.

Kim KY, Schumacher HR, Hunsche E, et al. A literature review of the epidemiology and treatment of acute gout. *Clin Ther.* 2003;25:1593–1617.

Richette P, Bardin T. Gout. *Lancet.* 2010;375:318–328.

Suresh E. Diagnosis and management of gout: A rational approach. *Postgrad Med J.* 2005;81:572–579.

Zhang W, Doherty M, Pascual E, et al. EULAR evidence based recommendations for gout. Parts I and II. *Ann Rheum Dis.* 2006;65:1301–1311.

III: Cancer- or Treatment-Related Symptoms

Hypercalcemia

Kimberson Tanco MD

Description

Hypercalcemia is a metabolic emergency and the most common paraneoplastic syndrome. Signs and symptoms of hypercalcemia may be subtle and can easily be missed unless there is a high index of suspicion. Symptoms depend on the rate of increase of calcium more so than the absolute level.

Epidemiology

- Hypercalcemia occurs in up to 30% of cancer patients and increases in frequency in advanced stages.
- It is more common in certain cancers, such as:
  - Squamous cell lung cancer
  - Breast cancer
  - Head and neck cancer
  - Myeloma
  - Renal cancer

Pathogenesis

- The regulation of calcium levels is centered on three key systems by:
  - Calcium absorption through the gastrointestinal tract
  - Renal excretion
  - Calcium resorption from the bone
- Three key mechanisms promote hypercalcemia of malignancy:
  - Parathyroid hormone-related protein
  - 1,25(OH)2D3
  - Lytic bone metastasis through cytokines, including IL-1, IL-6, and TNF-alpha

Clinical Features

- Neurologic:
  - Mood changes
  - Irritability
  - Delirium
  - Stupor
  - Coma
- Gastrointestinal effects:
  - Anorexia
  - Nausea
  - Vomiting
  - Constipation
  - Acute pancreatitis

- Renal manifestations:
  - Polyuria
  - Polydipsia
  - Nephrolithiasis
  - Renal insufficiency
- Cardiac effects:
  - May be fatal
  - Shortened QT
  - Bradycardia
  - Arrhythmias
  - Hypotension

Diagnosis

Differential diagnosis

- Malignancy: the most frequent cause of hypercalcemia in the hospital setting.
- Primary hyperparathyroidism is the most common cause in the community.
- Hypercalcemia of malignancy occurs suddenly, resulting in a faster increase in calcium levels and more symptomatic manifestations.
- Other potential causes include:
  - Granulomatous disorders, such as sarcoidosis
  - Medications that increase calcium levels, including hydrochlorothiazides and multivitamin supplements

Testing

- Measurement of serum ionized calcium is preferred over total serum calcium level. Total serum calcium level should be corrected for albumin level with the formulas below:
  - In Imperial Units:
    - corrected calcium (mg/dL) = serum calcium + 0.8 mg/dL (4 g/dL – serum albumin)
  - In SI Units:
    - corrected calcium (mmol/L) = serum calcium + 0.2 mmol/L (40 g/L – serum albumin)
- Parathyroid hormone-related protein is not routinely taken as it does not affect outcome; however, levels greater than 12 pmol/L may reflect bisphosphonate resistance.
- Levels of 1,25(OH)2D3 are elevated in granulomatous disorders such as sarcoidosis and lymphomas.

Treatment

Treatment of the underlying cancer and discontinuation of hypercalcemia-inducing medications are key.

- Aggressive intravenous rehydration with isotonic saline and close monitoring of volume status is the key initial step in treating hypercalcemia.
- Diuretics are no longer recommended, owing to risks of volume depletion and electrolyte imbalance.
- Calcitonin inhibits bone resorption and renal tubular calcium reabsorption and provides a quicker onset of action. However, its effect diminishes after 48 hours owing to tachyphylaxis due to down regulation of osteoclastic calcitonin receptors.
- Corticosteroids are used for steroid-responsive tumors such as lymphomas and myelomas.
- Bisphosphonates are the mainstay of treatment, particularly nitrogen-containing agents such as zoledronic acid.
  - Renal adverse effects can limit the use of bisphosphonates.
- Gallium nitrate may be considered in bisphosphonate-resistant cases.
  - Its long administration time and renal adverse effects can also limit its use.
- RANKL (receptor activator of nuclear factor kappa-B ligand) inhibitors include recombinant osteoprotegerin and denosumab. Their use in hypercalcemia of malignancy is promising but their cost is prohibitive.
- Antiparathyroid hormone-related protein antibodies have shown potential as more trials are being conducted.

Prognosis

- Hypercalcemia of malignancy is a poor prognostic indicator, with a median survival of 6 weeks.
- Treatment of hypercalcemia has not been shown to alter the disease course and improve the prognosis of the cancer.

Helpful Hints

- Hypercalcemia is the most common paraneoplastic condition but can be missed because symptoms may be subtle.
- Serum ionized calcium levels are the preferred laboratory measure. Otherwise, always remember to correct total serum calcium levels with serum albumin levels.
- Aggressive intravenous hydration is first line of treatment.
- Bisphosphonates are still the mainstay of treatment, although new novel treatments are currently being investigated.

Suggested Readings

Basso U, Maruzzo M, Roma A, et al. Malignant hypercalcemia. *Cur Med Chem.* 2011;18:3462–3467.

Legrand S. Modern management of malignant hypercalcemia. *Am J Hospice Palliat Med.* 2011;28:515–517.

Lumachi F, Brunello A, Roma A, et al. Medical treatment of malignancy-associated hypercalcemia. *Cur Med Chem.* 2008;15:415–421.

Lumachi F, Brunello A, Roma A, et al. Cancer-induced hypercalcemia. *Anticancer Res.* 2009;29:1551–1556.

III: Cancer- or Treatment-Related Symptoms

Lymphedema: Lower Extremity

Megan Bale Nelson MD

Definition

The accumulation of lymph outside the lymphatic system in a lower extremity, or both lower extremities. Lymphedema is an incurable but manageable lifelong condition.

Etiology/Types

- Primary lymphedema: An inherited condition of lymphatic system maldevelopment.
- Secondary lower extremity lymphedema: Occurs in cancer patients due to one, or a combination, of the following:
  - Cancer infiltration of lymph nodes
  - Lymph node surgical resection
  - Radiation-induced lymph node fibrosis
  - Bacterial and fungal infections
  - Lymphoproliferative diseases
  - Trauma
- Lower-extremity lymphedema is associated with the following cancers:
  - Pelvic or abdominal cancers such as prostate, testicular, cervical, uterine, ovarian, vulvar, colorectal, pancreatic, liver, or metastatic disease
  - Also occurs with cancers in the leg, such as melanoma or sarcomas
- Staging of lymphedema
  - Stage 0: Latent or subclinical condition in which edema is not evident despite impaired lymph transport. It may exist months or years before overt edema occurs.
  - Stage 1: The edema pits in response to pressure and is reduced significantly by elevation. There is no clinical evidence of fibrosis.
  - Stage 2: Edema does not pit in response to pressure and is not reduced by elevation. Moderate to severe fibrosis is evident on clinical examination.
  - Stage 3: Lymphedema is irreversible and develops as a result of repeated inflammatory insults. Fibrosis and sclerosis of the skin and subcutaneous tissues is present. This stage of edema is known also as lymphostatic elephantiasis.

Epidemiology

- Widely variable due to no internationally agreed upon definition of what constitutes lymphedema. However, overall risk of lymphedema for all cancers is reported to be 15.5%.

Risk Factors

- Extent or location of surgery
- Location of radiation
- Tumor obstruction
- Infection
- Weight gain
- Age
- Trauma history
- Chronic venous disease

Clinical Features

- Symptoms may arise days, weeks, months, or even years after cancer and its treatment.
  - A sense of fullness or heaviness
  - Swelling typically starts at the distal end of the extremity and progresses proximally. There is soft pitting edema initially.
  - Discomfort or pain in the leg
  - Clothing or shoes feel tighter
  - Weakness or decreased flexibility in the leg and/or ankle
  - Skin changes: In the early stages, skin may have a pinkish-red color and mildly elevated temperature due to increased vascularity. In the chronic stages, skin becomes thickened and exhibits areas of hyperkeratosis.
  - Stemmer's sign—epidermal tissues over the proximal phalanges of the feet become thickened
  - Loss of hair

Potential Complications of Lymphedema

- Increased risk of infection
- Difficulty healing wounds or infection
- Discomfort or pain
- Decreased lower extremity joint range of motion
- Impaired mobility and function
- Difficulty finding clothes and shoes to wear
- Psychological distress
- Lymphedema-induced lymphangiosarcoma, rare

Diagnosis

Investigation and workup depend on clinical presentation and may require a combination of the following:

- History and physical exam
- Circumferential measurements

- Water displacement
- Perometry
- Lymphoscintigraphy
- Bioimpedance spectroscopy
- Soft tissue imaging—MRI, CT, ultrasound
- It is important to rule out other potential causes of swelling, as indicated, which may include:
  - Blood clots
  - Tumor recurrence or metastases
  - Lipoedema
  - Heart failure
  - Hepatic or renal disease
  - Endocrine conditions
  - Medications
  - Hypoalbuminemia
  - Infections

Treatment
- Comprehensive decongestive therapy, including referral to a certified lymphedema therapist:
  - Manual lymphatic drainage
  - Compression garments
  - Bandaging
  - Avid skin and nail care
  - Exercise
- Extremity elevation when possible
- Intermittent pneumatic compression therapy
- Avoidance of temperature extremes
- Protective shoe wear
- Maintenance of a healthy weight
- Education of patient and caregivers

- Surgical interventions are available, including microsurgery, liposuction, and debulking; however, nonoperative management is the first-line treatment.

Helpful Hints
- Lower extremity lymphedema is associated with a wide range of cancer diagnoses.
- Other potential etiologies for swelling should be considered.
- Signs and symptoms of lymphedema may initially appear even years after cancer treatment.
- A comprehensive treatment approach is beneficial, including referral to a certified lymphedema therapist.
- Lifelong care for lower extremity lymphedema is required.

Suggested Readings
Davies R, Desborough S. Rehabilitation in cancer care. In: Rankin J, Robb K, Murtagh N, et al., eds. *Lymphoedema*. United Kingdom: Wiley-Blackwell; 2008:243–263.

Fu JB, Shin KY. Rehabilitation: Lymphedema. In: Kantarjian HM, Wolff RA, Koller CA, eds. *The MD Anderson Manual of Medical Oncology*. 2nd ed. China: McGraw-Hill; 2011:1359.

Keeley, V. Lymphoedema. In: Hanks G, Cherny NI, Christakis NA, et al. eds. *Oxford Textbook of Palliative Medicine*. 4th ed. New York, NY: Oxford University Press; 2010:972–982.

NLN Medical Advisory Committee. The Diagnosis and Treatment of Lymphedema. Retrieved from http://www.lymphnet.org/pdfDocs/nlntreatment.pdf. Last updated February 2011.

Strick, DM, Gamble GL. Cancer rehabilitation: Principles and practice. In: Stubblefield MD, O'Dell MW, eds. *Lymphedema in the Cancer Patient*. New York, NY: Demos Medical Publishing; 2009:1011–1022.

III: Cancer- or Treatment-Related Symptoms

Lymphedema: Upper Extremity

Jennifer Camp MD

Description

Lymphedema is abnormal swelling and accumulation of protein-rich lymphatic fluid in the soft tissues due to a disruption or blockage of lymphatic vessels by tumor, fibrosis, or inflammation. Upper extremity lymphedema is most often due to breast cancer and its treatments.

Etiology/Types

- Primary lymphedema is a rare developmental abnormality of the lymphatic system.
- Secondary lymphedema occurs as a result of cancer treatments, including surgical resection of lymphatic vessels and lymph nodes, mastectomy or breast conserving surgery without lymph node surgery, radiation-induced fibrosis, and obstruction by metastatic tumors.

Epidemiology

- Reports on the incidence of upper extremity lymphedema vary widely owing to a nonstandardized definition of lymphedema and degree of limb enlargement.
- One study found that patients who have been treated for breast cancer have a 15% to 20% chance of developing lymphedema.
- The risk of developing lymphedema is highest in women who have axillary lymph node dissection followed by radiation treatments.

Pathogenesis

- Lymph fluid is normally transported through a network of thin lymphatic vessels and lymph nodes, which ultimately empty into the venous system.
- When lymph fluid exceeds the system's transport capabilities, the protein-rich fluid accumulates in the soft tissues.
- These proteins increase the oncotic pressure and worsen edema.
- With time, the deposition of stagnant proteins leads to tissue fibrosis.
- Cellulitis, lymphangitis, and lymphatic valve incompetency are further complications that can worsen edema.

Risk Factors

- Axillary lymph node resection
- Radiation treatment
- Sentinel lymph node biopsy
- Obesity
- Slow healing of skin after surgery
- Older age
- Complex surgery
- Exercise does *not* cause lymphedema onset.

Clinical Features

- Stage 0—No swelling is evident, but there is a defect in the lymphatic system.
- Stage I—Pitting edema and a feeling of heaviness that subsides with limb elevation.
- Stage II—Nonpitting edema and the development of fibrotic tissue, which feels hard to palpation.
- Stage III—An extremely enlarged edematous limb with acanthotic skin and warty overgrowth; it is also known as elephantiasis and rarely occurs in breast cancer patients.
- The severity of lymphedema can also be described as minimal (less than 20% increase in volume), moderate (20%–40% increase), or severe (more than 40% increase) within each stage above.

Natural History

- If untreated, lymphedema can progress and become more difficult to manage.
- Severe lymphedema predisposes the patient to life-threatening complications, including infections and lymphangiosarcoma.

Diagnosis

Differential diagnosis

- Deep venous thrombosis
- Cellulitis/infection
- Malignancy
- Venous stasis
- Complex regional pain syndrome
- Chronic inflammatory arthritis
- Superior vena cava syndrome

History

- Insidious onset often after a minor injury or infection
- Patients report swelling, "heaviness," or "tightness" in the limb, decreased range of motion, difficulty fitting in clothing or wearing watches or bracelets, thickening of the skin, and numbness or paresthesias in the limb.

Examination

- Unilateral swelling, may be located in proximal and/or distal limb.
- Tissue fibrosis and skin changes
- Evaluate for any signs of infection, including redness, warmth, induration, or open wounds.

Testing

- Lymphoscintigraphy and MRI are no longer recommended tests for diagnosing lymphedema, but may be helpful tools for planning surgical intervention.
- Methods for measuring lymphedema include water displacement, tape measurement, infrared scanning, and bioelectrical impedance measures.
- The most widely used method is tape measurements at 4 points on both arms: the metacarpal–phalangeal joint, the wrist, 10 cm distal to the lateral epicondyle, and 15 cm proximal to the lateral epicondyle. Differences of 2 cm between arms are considered clinically significant.

Pitfalls

- There is no standardized test for measuring the affected limb, making it difficult to accurately assess lymphedema.

Red Flags

- The development of redness, warmth, induration, open skin wounds, fever, and malaise warrants immediate evaluation by a physician and treatment for cellulitis.

Treatment

Preventive

- Educate the patient and family.
- Teach good skin and nail hygiene.
- Avoid placing the limb in the dependent position.
- Elevate the affected limb when possible.
- Avoid tight clothing.
- Encourage frequent movement of the extremity.

Medical

- No pharmacologic therapy is recommended for lymphedema.
- Diuretics are ineffective.
- Antibiotics may be required on occasion to treat underlying infection.

Therapy

- Exercise: Aerobic exercise and weight lifting are safe.
- Complex decongestive therapy (CDT) with an experienced physical or occupational therapist: Includes manual lymph drainage, compressive wrapping with low-stretch bandages, compression garments (30–60 mmHg), skin and nail care, and exercises.
- The treatment phase of CDT typically lasts 2 to 4 weeks. After that, the maintenance phase includes a lifelong home-based program.
- Pneumatic compression pump
- Weight loss
- Laser therapy may decrease tissue fibrosis, stimulate macrophages, and encourage lymphangiogenesis.

Surgical

- Excisional procedures remove subcutaneous fat and fibrous tissue to the muscle fascia to promote lymph system communication between superficial and deep tissues.
- Physiologic microsurgical drainage procedures restore lymphatic flow and include lymphatic-to-lymphatic and lymphatic-to-venous anastomoses.
- Liposuction
- Superficial lymphangiectomy
- Fasciotomy
- Surgery is not routinely recommended for the treatment of lymphedema.

Consults

- Physical medicine and rehabilitation
- Physical or occupational therapy
- Plastic surgery
- Vascular surgery

Prognosis

- There is no cure for lymphedema. Treatments prevent worsening of the disease and the complications of the disease.
- Complications can be life threatening and include infection, septicemia, and lymphangiosarcoma.
- Poorly controlled lymphedema causes psychological distress and affects function and quality of life in cancer patients.

Helpful Hints

- In a patient who develops new and sudden onset of lymphedema, evaluation for other causes of swelling such as DVT should be considered.
- CDT is contraindicated for acute DVT, infection, active malignancy, and unwillingness or inability of the patient or family to participate in the program. Congestive heart failure is a relative contraindication.
- Avoid venous punctures, blood pressure cuff inflation, and any other trauma to a lymphedematous limb as it could worsen edema and/or lead to infection.

Suggested Readings

Guo Y, Truong AN. Rehabilitation of patients with breast cancer. In: Hunt KK, Robb GL, Strom EA, et al, eds. *Breast Cancer.* New York, NY: Springer Science + Business Media; 2008 485–504.

National Cancer Institute: PDQ® Lymphedema. Bethesda, MD: National Cancer Institute. Date last modified 6/30/2011. Available at: http://www.cancer.gov/cancertopics/pdq /supportivecare/lymphedema/healthprofessional. Accessed 10/26/2012.

Passik SD, McDonald MV. Psychosocial aspects of upper extremity lymphedema in women treated for breast carcinoma. *Cancer.* 1998;83(12 suppl):2817–2820.

Petrek JA, Pressman PI, Smith RA. Lymphedema: Current issues in research and management. *CA Cancer J Clin.* 2000;50(5):292–307.

Malnutrition

Carol Frankmann MS RD CSO LD CNSC

Description
Malnutrition is any disorder of nutrition status, including disorders resulting from deficiency of intake, impaired nutrient metabolism, or overnutrition.

Etiology/Types
- Undernutrition is malnutrition due to inadequate intake and/or reduced absorption of nutrients.
- Cancer cachexia is a complex syndrome characterized by progressive, involuntary weight loss, muscle wasting, anorexia, early satiety, fatigue, and anemia. The etiology is not entirely understood.

Epidemiology
- Weight loss, an indicator of malnutrition, ranges from 31% to 100% in cancer patients, depending on tumor site, stage, and treatment.
- Cachexia, observed in approximately 50% of cancer patients, is more common in patients with cancers of the lung, pancreas, upper gastrointestinal (GI) tract, and advanced disease.

Pathogenesis
- Nutritional status can be compromised by local effects of the tumor, tumor-induced alterations in metabolism, and/or the impact of treatment.
- Cancer cachexia is thought to be caused by a complex interaction between host neuroendocrine and cytokine systems, which promote systemic inflammation and tumor-derived products that promote direct tissue catabolism.

Risk Factors
- All cancer patients, especially those with aerodigestive tract or advanced disease
- Treatment that impacts the ability to ingest and/or absorb adequate nutrients.

Clinical Features
- Unintentional weight loss of 10% in 6 months or body mass index (BMI) of less than 18.5
- Impaired ability to ingest or absorb nutrients
- Decreased functional capacity
- Delayed wound healing

Natural History
- Malnutrition leads to increased susceptibility to infection, delayed wound healing, impairment of physical and cognitive function, detrimental effects on every organ, and eventually death if not reversed.

Diagnosis
- All patients with cancer should undergo nutritional screening to identify those who require comprehensive nutrition assessment and a plan of care.
- The Patient Generated Subjective Global Assessment is a validated screening tool specifically for cancer patients.

Differential diagnosis
- Malnutrition/undernutrition, cancer cachexia.

History
- Change in weight, height
- Diet/nutrient intake
- Presence of symptoms that impact nutrition, such as anorexia, nausea, vomiting, diarrhea, constipation, stomatitis, mucositis, dysphagia, alterations in taste and smell, pain, depression, and anxiety.
- Level of activity and function

Examination
- Weight, height, BMI
- Decreased subcutaneous tissue
- Skeletal muscle loss, temporal wasting
- Edema, ascites
- Oral cavity, dentition, swallowing
- GI tract function
- Skin, hair, and nail changes; presence of pressure sore, open wound, fistula

Testing
- Serum albumin, prealbumin, transferrin
- Handgrip dynamometry

Pitfalls
- Hepatic transport proteins (albumin, prealbumin, transferrin) often decrease in response to metabolic stress rather than changes in nutrient intake, so laboratory results should be evaluated in conjunction with weight history, medical condition, and nutrient intake in cancer patients.

Red Flags
- Malnourished surgical patients are at increased risk for postoperative morbidity and mortality.
- Aggressive feeding in malnourished patients can lead to respiratory and cardiac failure associated with a refeeding syndrome marked by hypophosphatemia, hypokalemia, and hypomagnesemia. Nutrition support should be initiated cautiously in malnourished patients, beginning below nutrient needs and progressing slowly over 7 to 10 days and while monitoring organ function, fluid balance, serum electrolytes, and glucose daily.

Treatment
- Oral diet should be used for patients with normal GI function who are able to consume adequate amounts of food and/or enteral nutrition supplements. Modifications in diet may be needed to aid in the management of symptoms that impact nutrient intake.
- Nutrition support therapy, such as enteral/parenteral nutrition, is appropriate for patients receiving active anticancer treatment who are malnourished and anticipated to be unable to ingest and/or absorb adequate nutrients for a prolonged period of time.
- Enteral nutrition should be used in patients with good GI function when oral intake is inadequate to meet nutrition requirements.
  - Nasogastric (NG), nasoduodenal, or nasojejunal enteral feedings are best for short-term support of less than 2 weeks.
  - Percutaneous endoscopic gastrostomy (PEGs) and percutaneous endoscopic jejunostomy tubes (PEJs) are for longer-term feedings.
- Parenteral nutrition should only be used in malnourished patients with impaired GI function who are expected to be unable to ingest and/or absorb adequate nutrients for at least 7 to 14 days.

Complications of treatment
- Enteral nutrition increases the risk of aspiration, sinusitis, or nasoesophageal erosion from NG tube.
- Parenteral nutrition is associated with an increased risk of infection and the potential for glucose, electrolyte, and fluid abnormalities.

Contraindications for enteral and parenteral nutrition support
- Enteral nutrition should not be used with impaired GI function, severe diarrhea, intractable vomiting, or GI fistulas that are difficult to bypass with an enteral tube. Patients with mucositis, esophagitis, and/or infections in the mouth or throat may not be able to tolerate the presence of an NG tube.
- Parenteral nutrition should not be used routinely in patients undergoing major surgery, as an adjunct to chemotherapy, or in patients undergoing head and neck, abdominal, or pelvic irradiation.
- Palliative use of nutrition support therapy in terminally ill cancer patients is rarely indicated.

Prognosis
- Some patients with cachexia respond to nutrition therapy, but most will not see a significant reversal of the syndrome. Appetite stimulants are minimally effective.
- Provision of adequate nutrition is effective in restoring nutritional status in cancer patients in the absence of cachexia.
- In addition to adequate nutrition, physical activity is necessary to increase lean body mass and improve functional status.

Helpful Hint
- Proactive nutrition screening, assessment, and intervention are essential in reducing malnutrition and its adverse impact on morbidity and mortality.

Suggested Readings
August DA, Huhmann MB, ASPEN Board of Directors. A.S.P.E.N. Clinical Guidelines: Nutrition support therapy during adult anticancer treatment and in hematopoetic cell transplantation. *J Parenter Enteral Nutr.* 2009;33:472–500.

Marian M, Roberts S, eds. *Clinical Nutrition for Oncology Patients.* Sudbury, MA: Jones and Bartlett; 2010.

National Cancer Institute at the National Institutes of Health. Nutrition in cancer care (PDQ®). http://www.cancer.gov /cancertopics/pdq/supportivecare/nutrition/Health Professional, accessed February 12, 2013.

Mastectomy: Reconstruction Concerns

Ying Guo MD MS

Description
When breast conservation treatment is not recommended, mastectomy, followed by surgical reconstruction, can provide the patient with aesthetically acceptable results.

Epidemiology
- Over 226,000 new cases of breast cancer in the United States in 2012
- Shoulder restriction has been reported in under 1% to 67% of patients with early breast cancer following surgery and radiation treatment.
- Lymphedema has been reported in 0% to 34%.
- Shoulder/arm pain has been reported in 9% to 68%.
- Arm weakness reported in 9% to 28%.
- 6% to 23% of patients demonstrate deficits in trunk function following transverse rectus abdominis muscle (TRAM) reconstruction.

Pathophysiology
- Scar tissue in the surgical site and in radiated tissue can lead to kyphosis and a protracted shoulder posture.

Risk Factors
- Irradiated patients have slightly increased odds of lymphedema and shoulder restriction compared with nonirradiated patients.

Clinical Features
- Physical function may be impaired depending on the degree of muscle that is sacrificed, denervated, or injured in creating flaps for breast reconstruction.
- Tightness due to removal of muscle and associated tissue
- Contracture and fear of movement can lead to decreased range of motion.
- Decreased abdominal function can hinder the patient's ability to perform sit-ups, and getting-out-of-bed activities.
- For patients who receive perforator flaps, the majority are able to return to preoperative activity in 3 to 6 months.

Diagnosis

History
- More aggressive surgery with postoperative radiation will likely have greater adverse effects on the patient's function.
- The type of reconstruction varies:
  - Immediate reconstruction versus delayed reconstruction
  - Implant versus autologous tissue
  - Pedicled TRAM flap—transverse rectus abdominus myocutaneous flap
  - Latissimus dorsi (LD) flap is usually transferred to the mastectomy site as a pedicled flap.
  - Free TRAM flap
  - The transverse upper gracilis (TUG) flap uses skin and soft tissue along with blood vessel supply.
  - The deep inferior epigastric perforator (DIEP) flap uses fat and skin from the abdominal area.

Examination
- Range of motion of upper extremity, spine
- Strength of trunk, upper extremity

Treatment
- To restore function of the whole person:
  - Physical therapy and occupational therapy
  - Stretching and strengthening of affected soft tissue, yoga
  - Treat lymphedema
  - Counseling and support groups

Prognosis
- Outpatient therapy is effective in improving range of motion (ROM), balance, and posture.

Helpful Hints
- Pain is severe after implants for 3 to 4 weeks, and 6 to 8 weeks after flap surgery.

III: Cancer- or Treatment-Related Symptoms

■ Three months after surgery and complete healing of the incision site, a more aggressive range of motion, exercise, and deep tissue massage program around the scar area can be prescribed.

■ Women who have undergone mastectomy with or without reconstruction need time to adjust. These patients will also benefit from support groups and additional counseling, if necessary.

Suggested Readings

Atisha D, Alderman AK. A systematic review of abdominal wall function following abdominal flaps for postmastectomy breast reconstruction. *Ann Plast Surg.* 2009;63(2):222.

Hamdi M, Weiler-Mithoff EM, Webster MH. Deep inferior epigastric perforator flap in breast reconstruction: Experience with the first 50 flaps. *Plast Reconstr Surg.* 1999;103(1):86.

Lee TS, Kilbreath SL, Refshauge KM, et al. Prognosis of the upper limb following surgery and radiation for breast cancer. *Breast Cancer Res Treat.* 2008;110(1):19–37.

Mastectomy: Treatment Complications

Ying Guo MD MS

Description
Mastectomy can cause both physical and psychological impairment.

Etiology/Type
- Breast surgery type:
  - Lumpectomy: removes the breast lump and a margin of tissue around the lump. It is a breast-conserving surgery.
  - Partial mastectomy: removes part of the breast that contains the tumor and some surrounding tissue.
  - Mastectomy: removes the whole breast.
  - Modified radical mastectomy: removes the whole breast, along with some of the lymph nodes under the arm, and often the lining over the chest muscles.
  - Radical mastectomy: removes the whole breast, lymph nodes, and the pectoralis major muscle.

Epidemiology
- One of every eight women in the United States will develop breast cancer in their lifetime.
- Roughly 2.5 million women in the United States are survivors of breast cancer.
- Late sequelae post mastectomy:
  - Pain (12%–51%)
  - Impairments in range of motion (ROM; 2%–51%)
  - Edema (6%–43%)
  - Decreased muscle strength (17%–33%)
  - Lymphedema (8%–56%)
  - Sexual dysfunction (12% after surgery)

Pathophysiology
- Postoperative scar tissue formation
- Radiation-induced fibrosis
- Protective posturing, causing shoulder protraction
- Pain

Risk Factors
- Women with lymphedema have greater upper extremity impairment and limitation in activities than women without.
- Shoulder range of motion is limited in up to 45% of patients who have sentinel node biopsy, and in 86% of patients who have undergone axillary clearance.

Clinical Features
- Local inflammation, postoperative pain, limited limb use due to pain, altered posture secondary to pain and contractures.
- Early sequelae: may vary depending on surgical procedure, type of reconstruction.
  - Pain:
    - Postmastectomy pain
    - Presence of widespread pressure, hyperalgesia, and myofascial trigger points (TrPs) in neck and shoulder muscles
  - Decrease in shoulder range of motion
  - Seroma
  - Infection
  - Psychosocial impact:
    - Body image
    - Feelings of unattractiveness
- Late sequelae:
  - Pain, including intercostal and brachial involvement
  - Impairments in range of motion
  - Edema
  - Decreased muscle strength
  - Lymphedema (Chapter 36).
  - Sexual dysfunction
- Difficulty washing or combing hair, difficulty reaching items
- Decrease in strength from disuse
- Poor posture
- Back pain

Diagnosis

Differential diagnosis
- Frozen shoulder
- A/C (acromioclavicular) joint dysfunction

History
- Decreased shoulder range of motion: gradual onset, usually postsurgery
- Disuse weakness
- Poor posture: kyphosis, shoulder protraction

Examination
- Range of motion of the shoulder
- Scar tissue
- Presence of trigger points in neck, shoulder, spine, and pectoralis area

Treatment

- Stretching and strengthening program
- Treatment of lymphedema
- Support group

Prognosis

- Outpatient therapy is effective in improving ROM, posture, and function.

Helpful Hints

- Encourage patients to use their upper extremities.

- Weight-lifting limitations are no longer recommended; supervised weight training is encouraged.
- Go to www.lymphnet.org for a list of lymphedema-certified therapists.

Suggested Reading

Leidenius M, Leppänen E, Krogerus L, von Smitten K. Motion restriction and axillary web syndrome after sentinel node biopsy and axillary clearance in breast cancer. *Am J Surg.* 2003;185(2):127–130.

Mental Health: Behavioral Disorders

An Ngo DO ■ Alan Valentine MD

Description

Approximately 50% of cancer patients have psychological and emotional difficulties. Prompt diagnosis of psychological distress is essential, as functional progress in a rehabilitation program is often hindered when patients have high levels of distress.

Adjustment Disorder

- Most prevalent psychiatric disorder in cancer patients
- Characterized by emotional or behavioral changes (sadness and/or anxiety) attributed to a stressful event.
- Onset is within 3 months of the triggering event and does not persist beyond 6 months of termination of the stressor.
- Treatment: Brief psychotherapy (focus on immediate problems and coping skills), support groups, and formal group therapy.

Depression

- Higher rates in patients with advanced cancers
- Cancers with increased incidence of depression: lung, breast, head and neck, and pancreas
- Most reliable symptoms: guilt, loss of self-esteem, feelings of hopelessness, worthlessness, and wishing to die
- Treatment: combination of supportive psychotherapy, antidepressant medications, support groups, and cognitive behavioral techniques
- Pharmacological interventions are the mainstay for treatment of cancer patients with moderate to severe depression.
  - Patients with insomnia: Recommend using a sedating antidepressant such as mirtazapine.
  - Patients with poor pain control: Use a combination of serotonin and norepinephrine modulator (venlafaxine or duloxetine). May consider a tricyclic antidepressant (TCA).
  - Use selective serotonin receptor inhibitors (SSRIs) for patients with serious medical illnesses or in the elderly to minimize side effects.
  - Almost all antidepressants may lower the seizure threshold—avoid bupropion.
  - Consider psychostimulants to treat concomitant fatigue and to increase alertness.

Anxiety

- Symptoms: worry, restlessness, jitteriness, tension, vigilance, distractibility, insomnia, autonomic hyperactivity, diaphoresis, shortness of breath, or numbness
- Etiology: may be a component of a generalized disorder: adjustment disorder, generalized anxiety disorder, or panic disorder. May also be present in delirium.
- Rule out medical issues or medications that may be causing the patient's anxiety.
  - Pain is a very common cause of anxiety. Anxiety levels decrease with adequate pain control.
- Treatment: psychotherapy and anxiolytic medications; brief psychotherapy may be helpful in crisis-related issues.
- Consultant to provide psychotherapy: increase the patient's sense of self-worth; explore issues of separation and loss via hypnosis, relaxation, and imagery-guided therapy
- Pharmacological treatment: SSRIs may be used for generalized anxiety disorder or for panic disorder. May need a short-acting benzodiazepine until the antidepressant takes effect.

Delirium

- Symptoms: disturbance of level of consciousness, disorientation, fluctuation of emotion, impaired memory, and alteration of sleep–wake cycle
  - Waxing and waning symptoms
  - Reversible process
- One of the most frequent neuropsychiatric complications in patients with advanced cancer; incidence of 15% to 75%.
- Delirium is a significant cause of distress for the patient and for their caregivers.
- Etiology: direct effects of cancer on the central nervous system (CNS) or indirectly due to medical complications/effects of treatments
- Chemotherapy agents that may cause delirium: methotrexate, fluorouracil, vincristine, vinblastine, bleomycin, cisplatin, asparaginase, procarbazine, corticosteroids, and ifosfamide.

- Dementia has very similar clinical features. In dementia patients, there is a more insidious or progressive onset, short-term memory impairments initially, and patients usually have a clear sensorium.
- Treatment: Correct underlying medical factors (electrolytes, nutrition). Employ supportive measures: quiet and well-lit room, familiar faces and objects, clock/calendar.
  - Antipsychotics: Haloperidol, risperidone, olanzapine, quetiapine

Functional Impact of Behavior Disorders
- Decreased motivation, apathy, anxiety, and/or hopelessness may interfere with patients' ability to participate in a rehabilitation program.
- Depressed patients make slower functional progress, are unable to achieve rehabilitation goals, and thus, have increased length of stays.
- These patients are less likely to seek and complete outpatient rehabilitation programs.
- Ultimately, in order for patients to achieve adequate functional return, behavioral distress needs to be managed appropriately.

Prognosis for Behavior Disorders
- With the appropriate psychological and psychopharmacological regimen, treatment of behavioral disorders is effective and can lead to improvement of quality of life for cancer patients.

Helpful Hints
- Use a screening tool such as the Edmonton Symptom Assessment System or the Hospital Anxiety and Depression Scale to quickly identify those in need of psychosocial interventions.
- Early referral to a psychiatric specialist

Suggested Readings
Braun I, Valentine A. Depression, anxiety, and delirium. In: Pazdur R, Wagman LD, Camphausen KA, Hoskins WJ, eds. *Cancer Management: A Multidisciplinary Approach.* Norwalk, CT: UBM Medica; 2009:905–915.

Chochinov HM. Depression in cancer patients. *Lancet Oncol.* 2001;2:499–505.

Li M, Fitzgerald P, Rodin G. Evidence-based treatment of depression in patients with cancer. *J Clin Oncol.* 2012;30(11):1187–1196.

Traeger L, Greer JA, Fernandez-Robles C, et al. Evidence-based treatment of anxiety in patients with cancer. *J Clin Oncol.* 2012;30(11):1197–1205.

Mental Health: Depression

Karina Ramirez MD ■ Maxine De La Cruz MD

Description
Patients with cancer have a high rate of psychiatric comorbidities. Generally these comorbidities manifest in the form of adjustment disorder, depressed mood, clinical depression, and anxiety disorder. It is important for clinicians to be able to recognize the above conditions to be able to initiate treatment options early.

Etiology
The cancer patient can undergo a lot of psychological stress throughout the process of investigation of a physical diagnosis of cancer and initiation of individualized treatment.
- During the diagnosis phase, patients can experience a considerable amount of fear as they prepare for the possibility of the start of a serious illness.
- After the diagnosis, many patients experience a sense of shock or feeling numb, which can lead to increased episodes of anxiety.
- During the active phase of treatment, patients have to cope with cancer pain and the side effects of active therapies, which can tax their psychological resources.
- Patients begin to experience loss of physical integrity, changes in family and social roles, and increased dependence on others and on the medical system.
- All of these serve as sources of chronic mental strain, which can lead patients to develop symptoms of clinical depression and anxiety.

Epidemiology
- Age of onset of depression is variable.
- Male-to-female ratio of depression is similar.
- Risk of depression is higher if there is a positive family history.
- Prevalence studies on depressive disorders among cancer patients show a wide variation of between 1% and 30%.

Risk Factors
- Gender: In the normal population, females have a higher incidence than males. In advanced cancer patients, males are classified as more seriously depressed.
- Age: more common in younger patients (less than 45 years of age) than in older adults.
- Prior history of depression: Life-threatening illness is a major stressor that can precipitate depression to recur.
- Social support: Poor social support leads to more episodes of depression.
- Functional status: Patients with advanced disease with loss of independence and decline in functional status can trigger increased distress and onset of depression symptoms.
- Pain: Uncontrolled pain leads to higher risk of depression.
- Illness: cancers that metastasize to brain, pituitary tumors that lead to hypercortisolism or Cushing's syndrome, pancreatic cancer diagnosis
- Treatment-related factors: corticosteroids, chemotherapy (vincristine, vinblastine, asparagines, intrathecal methotrexate, interferon, interleukin), and radiotherapy
- Existential distress: When one is facing a life-threating crisis, existential issues of legacy, meaning of life, maintenance of dignity and self-control, and concerns over the welfare of other family members can elicit symptoms of depression.

Diagnosis

Differential diagnosis
- Adjustment disorder with depressed mood: Patients have a known stressor that causes a reaction similar to depressive episode, but the reaction is triggered specifically by that stressor.
- Anhedonia: loss of interest or pleasure in almost all activities
- Dysthymic disorder: patients with "low-level depression" that lasts at least 2 years
- Anxiety disorders: generalized anxiety disorder, posttraumatic stress disorder, obsessive compulsive disorder
- Medical conditions: hypothyroidism, anemia, Parkinson's disease, cancer
- Substance-induced mood disorders: illicit drugs, B-blockers, glucocorticoids, benzodiazepines

DSM-IV criteria

- Must have depressed mood, loss of interest or pleasure, weight loss or gain, insomnia or hypersomnia, psychomotor agitation or retardation, fatigue or loss of energy, feelings of worthlessness or excessive or inappropriate guilt, decreased concentration, and recurrent thoughts of death or suicidal ideation or planning or a suicide attempt.

Treatment

Supportive

- Recognize the patient as a "whole person"
- Initiate supportive psychotherapy using active listening and supportive verbal interventions.
- Psychosocial therapy: psychotherapy, group psychotherapy, hypnotherapy, psychoeducation, relaxation and biofeedback techniques, self-help groups, and cognitive-behavioral therapy

Pharmacologic

- Factors such as prognosis and time frame for treatment play an important role in determining type of pharmacotherapy for depression.
  - Patients with several months to live: choose medications that can take 4 weeks for response versus actively dying patient: choose rapid acting psychostimulant.

Tricyclic Antidepressants (TCA)

- Tertiary amines (amitriptyline, doxepin, imipramine)
  - Greater propensity for side effects
  - Blockade of muscarinic cholinergic receptors, alpha-adrenergic blockades lead to hypotension, H1 histamine receptor blockade sedation and drowsiness, which can lead to increased fall risk
- Secondary amines (nortriptyline, desipramine)
  - In cancer patients, fewer side effects and better tolerated
  - Side effects: constipation, dry mouth, urinary retention, serious tachycardia or arrhythmias
  - Start low doses 10 to 25 mg qhs (nightly) and increase in 10- to 25-mg increments q2 to 4 days, often to doses in range of 25 to 125 mg in cancer patients versus 150 to 300 mg in general population.
- Use amitriptyline, doxepin in patients with insomnia and agitation as more sedating.
- Therapeutic response reached in 3 to 6 weeks. Don't use if complicated cardiac or medical history or if patient has a short life expectancy.

Selective Serotonin Reuptake Inhibitors (SSRIs)

- SSRIs such as bupropion, fluoxetine, paroxetine, fluvoxamine, and sertraline.

- Safer and fewer side effects than TCAs
- Side effects: increased intestinal motility, loose stools, nausea/vomiting, insomnia, headaches, sexual dysfunction, anxiety, tremor, restlessness, and akathisia
- All SSRIs inhibit hepatic isoenenzymes; most potent are Paxil and Luvox.
- Fluoxetine (Prozac) and its active metabolite norfluoxetine have long half-life of elimination. When stopped it takes 5 weeks to wash out effect.
- Side effects: increased anxiety, weight loss, and mild nausea
- Reach steady state in 5 to 6 weeks.
- Bupropion increases risk of seizures

Serotonin–Norepinephrine Reuptake Inhibitors (SNRIs)

- SNRIs such as venlafaxine (Effexor), duloxetine (Cymbalta), desvenlafaxine (Pristiq)

Duloxetine (Cymbalta)

- Metabolized by liver. Do not use in patients with liver dysfunction.
- Side effects: Gastrointestinal (GI), which includes nausea, vomiting, dry mouth, and constipation/diarrhea. Somnolence (prescribe qhs), less common sexual side effects versus SSRIs.
- Can be used as adjuvant, especially in patients with concomitant neuropathic type pain.
- Start at 20 mg twice a day. Can increase to 60 mg a day.

Venlafaxine (Effexor)

- Metabolized by liver, excreted by kidney
- Start 37.5 mg q12 hours and increase to 75 mg q6 hours; maximum dose 375 mg/24 hours
- Side effects: nausea, dizziness, sedation, constipation, increased risk of GI bleed

Mirtazapine (Remeron)

- A tetracyclic compound unrelated to TCAs
- Mechanism of action: blocks pre- and postsynaptic alpha-2 receptors and serotonin receptors 5HT2 and 5HT3 with low affinity for alpha-1 receptor.
- Side effects: sedation even at low doses, weight gain, and increase in appetite (use as appetite stimulant) and dry mouth, less sexual dysfunction
- Starting doses 15 to 30 mg daily and can be increased to 30 to 45 mg in 1- to 2-week intervals.

Trazadone

- Antidepressant—at doses of 100 to 300 mg/day
- High affinity for alpha1-adrenoreceptors leads to orthostatic hypotension.

- Side effects: sedating and drowsiness; use in cancer patients with insomnia.
- Use as adjuvant for analgesic effect if both pain and depression present.
- Leads to arrhythmias in patients with cardiac disease
- Priapism: caution use in men.

Heterocyclic antidepressants
- Maprotiline, amoxapine
- Side effects like TCAs
- Maprotiline: avoid in patients with brain tumors or seizure disorder.
- Amoxapine: has mild dopamine-blocking effects so in combination with antiemetics can lead to extrapyramidal symptoms/dyskinesias.

Monoamine oxidase inhibitors
Isocarboxazid, phenelzine, tranylcypromine
- Less desired in cancer patients owing to interaction and side effect profile.
- Interactions with food rich in tyramine
- Interactions with other medications: psychostimulants, phenylpropranolamine, and pseudoephedrine
- Can lead to hypertensive crisis and development of strokes and death.
- In combination with opioids, leads to myoclonus and delirium.

Psychostimulants
Dextroamphetamine, methylphenidate, pemoline
- Rapid onset of action
- More helpful in treatment of depression in cancer patients with advanced disease. Use in patients with dysphoric symptoms, psychomotor retardation, and mild cognitive impairments.
- Benefit:
  - Helps with fatigue symptoms by increasing energy.
  - Improve attention, concentration
  - Low doses: stimulate appetite, promote a sense of well-being
  - Helps reduce sedation secondary to opioids.

Methylphenidate
- Dose: start low 2.5 mg po q8am and noon (max dose 30 mg/day) and increase slowly until desired effect or side effects.
- Side effects: nervousness, overstimulation, anxiety, increased blood pressure, increased heart rate, tremor, paranoia, insomnia, confusion
- Use short term: 1 to 2 months; 2/3 can be weaned off without recurrence, if recurrent depression can use for 1 year with less concern for abuse.

Pemoline
- Less potent, less potential of abuse, does not require triplicate prescription
- Comes in chewable tablet: used in patients who can't swallow
- Start at 18.75 mg q8am and noon, increase gradually (75 mg/24 hours)
- Caution in liver dysfunction; monitor liver function test

Alprazolam
- Benzodiazepine, good in patients with anxiety and depression; starting dose of 0.25 mg q8 hours (range 4–6 mg daily)
- Caution in elderly patients as increased risk of falls and associated complications with hip fractures and risk of abuse potential

Olanzapine (Zyprexa)
- Exact mechanism of action unknown but antagonizes dopamine, serotonin 5-HT2, and other receptors
- Metabolized by liver
- Side effects: dizziness, somnolence, extrapyramidal symptoms, weight gain, and appetite stimulation
- Can be used for anxiety and depression to improve moods.
- Dosing: 2.5 mg po qhs and increase gradually

Electroconvulsive therapy
- Often reserved for medication-resistant depression
- Especially useful in the elderly

Helpful Hints
- Best outcome for treatment of depression is both psychotherapy and pharmacological therapy.
- Underdiagnosis and undertreatment of depression in the dying patient can lead to suffering and poor quality of life.

Suggested Readings
Rosenfeld B, Abbey J, Pessin H. Depression and hopelessness near the end of life: Assessment and treatment. In: Werth J, Blevings D, eds. *Psychosocial Issues Near the End of Life: A Resource for Professional Care Providers.* Washington, DC: American Psychological Association; 2006:163–182.

Strong V, Waters R, Hibberd C, et al. Management of depression in people with cancer (Smart Oncology 1): A randomized trial: *Lancet.* 2008;372:340.

Wilson KG. Diagnosis and management of depression in palliative care. In: Chochinov H, Breitbart W, eds. *Handbook of Psychiatry in Palliative Medicine.* New York, NY: Oxford University Press; 2000:25–49.

III: Cancer- or Treatment-Related Symptoms

Pain: Conservative Management

Ahsan Azhar MD FACP ■ Suresh K. Reddy MD FFARCS

Description
- Cancer pain occurs in up to 70% of patients with advanced cancer.
- It tends to be one of the most common symptoms, both during active treatment as well as in the terminal phases of cancer.

Types of Cancer Pain
- Cancer pain is of two types:
  - Nociceptive
  - Neuropathic

Treatment of Cancer Pain
- Treatment of cancer pain includes:
  - Pharmacological treatment with opioids and nonopioids
  - Nonpharmacological treatment, including anesthetic blocks, neurosurgical procedures, cognitive-behavioral therapy, acupuncture, massage, and physical and occupational therapy

Pharmacological Treatment
- Pain can be controlled with a simple, stepwise approach using the World Health Organization (WHO) analgesic ladder model.
- Strength of analgesic agent to be used is based on the severity of pain.
- Selection of the adjuvant agent is based on the pathophysiology of the underlying process.

Opioid analgesics
- Weak opioids include codeine, hydrocodone (oral, in combination with acetaminophen), and tramadol.
- Strong opioids include morphine (the most commonly used), oxycodone, hydromorphone, methadone, oxymorphone, and fentanyl.
- Tapentadol has both opioid and nonopioid properties (mu-opioid receptor agonist as well as norepinephrine reuptake inhibitor properties).
- Choice of opioid is based on:
  - Patient's general condition
  - Type of pain
  - Severity of pain
  - Underlying renal and liver functions

- Oral route is preferred, but intravenous route can be used for refractory pain. Rectal and subcutaneous routes can also be used with most of the agents with nearly 100% bioavailability.

Titration of opioid analgesics
- In opioid-naïve patients, weaker opioids are started and are titrated as needed.
- If pain is not controlled, then a stronger opioid is initiated.
- Initially, a short-acting opioid is used, and then a sustained release formulation may be introduced.
- Provision should be given to cover breakthrough pain. A short-acting opioid may be used for breakthrough pain with a dose of 10% to 15% of total daily opioid dose.

Side effects of opioid analgesics
- Common side effects include:
  - Constipation
  - Drowsiness (opioid induced sedation)
  - Itching
  - Nausea
- Serious side effects include:
  - Opioid-induced neurotoxicity
    - May range from slight uneasiness, agitation or restlessness, vivid dreams, myoclonic jerks, visual and auditory hallucinations to overt confusion and delirium.
    - Can be prevented by avoiding concomitant use of multiple opioids as well as other medications which can cause sedation and confusion.
    - Can be managed with reducing the dose of or rotating the opioid, hydrating the patient, and correcting constipation aggressively. Addition of haloperidol can help control the agitation and restlessness.
  - Respiratory depression
- Tolerance develops to most of the common side effects except for constipation.

Management of side effects of opioid analgesics
- Opioid-induced nausea: can be managed by the addition of a simple antiemetic such as metoclopramide, as scheduled.

- Opioid-induced sedation: usually diminishes, but if persistent can be managed with the addition of psychostimulants such as methylphenidate.
- Opioid-induced constipation: over 90% of patients on opioid analgesics never develop tolerance to constipation. A daily scheduled bowel regimen with the addition of a stimulant laxative must be added.
- Opioid rotation or switching is used to rapidly correct severe toxicity from these agents.
- Opioid equianalgesic dose tables aide in the switch of opioids. Dose reduction by 30% to 50% should be done to account for incomplete cross tolerance among opioid analgesics (see Table 42.1).

Nonopioid analgesics
- Acetaminophen can be used for mild body aches and pains. Caution should be exercised, as acetaminophen has the potential for liver injury.
- Nonsteroidal anti-inflammatory drugs can be used for bone metastatic pain and other musculoskeletal pain syndromes. Caution should be used with renal failure, gastrointestinal ulcerations, and heart failure.

Adjuvant medications
- *Anticonvulsants* such as carbamazepine, gabapentin, and pregabalin may be used for neuropathic pain.
- *Tricyclic antidepressants* such as amitriptyline can also be used for neuropathic pain.
- *Bisphosphonates* can be used for bony pain from metastasis and for the prevention of pathological fractures.
- *Corticosteroids* are useful for bone pain or when inflammation is the underlying problem.

Nonpharmacological Treatment
- *Anesthetic procedures* include celiac plexus block, vertebroplasty, and neuroaxial opioid instillation.
- *Cordotomy* may be useful in refractory pain syndromes.
- Relaxation techniques, cognitive-behavioral techniques, physical modalities, massage therapy, and acupuncture are useful adjuvants to control pain.

Table 42.1   Commonly Used Opioids With Equianalgesic Ratios

Drug	Usual starting dosages
Full Opioid Agonists	
Codeine	15–30 mg orally every 3–4 hours
Propoxyphene	100 mg orally every 4–6 hours
Tramadol	50 mg orally every 4–6 hours
Morphine	15–30 mg orally every 3–4 hours
	30–60 mg orally every 8–12 hours
Hydromorphone	2–4 mg orally every 4–6 hours
Transdermal Fentanyl	25–50 mcg/hr transdermal every 3 days
Oxycodone	5–10 mg orally every 3–4 hours
Methadone	5–10 mg orally every 8–12 hours
	2.5–5 mg orally every 3–4 hours for breakthrough pain

Morphine can be given as an immediate release formulation or as a sustained release preparation. (It is recommended that an agent with relatively rapid onset such as immediate release morphine be provided to patients who take sustained release morphine, to provide rescue medication for breakthrough pain.)

Equianalgesic dosing table

	From same parenteral opioid to oral opioid	From oral opioid to oral morphine	From oral morphine to oral opioid
Codeine	NA	0.15	10–15
Morphine	3	1	1
Oxycodone	NA	1.5	0.7
Hydromorphone	3	5	0.2
Methadone	1–2	10–15	0.1–0.15

Source: *The MD Anderson Supportive and Palliative Care Handbook*. 4th ed. 2008.

III: Cancer- or Treatment-Related Symptoms

Some Key Concepts

- Tolerance to opioid analgesics is a physiological state characterized by a decrease in effect of a medication owing to its chronic administration.
- Physical dependence develops with chronic use of opioids when the body becomes physiologically adapted to the presence of opioids. Rapid reduction in dose may lead to withdrawal symptoms.
- Addiction (psychological dependence) is an aberrant behavior of seeking or craving for a drug for nonmedical reasons, despite harm.
- Pseudoaddiction can result from undertreatment of pain, where the patient will ask for pain medication frequently. This can be misinterpreted as addiction.

Helpful Hints

- Efforts must be made to identify the underlying mechanism of the pain syndrome.
- WHO ladder should be kept in mind while initiating treatment for pain.
- Opioids should not be withheld and should be introduced early for prompt relief of cancer pain.

- Scheduled antiemetics and laxatives (bowel regimen) should be added at the time of initiating opioid treatment.
- Patients should be regularly monitored for developing signs of opioid induced neurotoxicity.
- Opioid rotation must be carried out for managing opioid-induced neurotoxicity.
- Adjuvant medications and nonpharmacological techniques should also be introduced where appropriate.

Suggested Readings

Hanks G, Cherny NI, Christakis NA, et al. eds. *Oxford Textbook of Palliative Medicine* (chap 10.1). 4th ed. New York, NY: Oxford University Press; 2009.

NCCN Guidelines for Adult Cancer Pain Management. Version 2.2012. http://www.nccn.org/professionals/physician_gls /f_guidelines.asp#age

WHO. *Cancer Pain Relief and Palliative Care*. 2nd ed. Geneva: WHO; 1996.

Zech DF, Gound S, Lynch J, et al. Validation of WHO guidelines for cancer pain relief: 10 year prospective study. *Pain*. 1995;63:65–76.

Pain: Interventional Techniques

Brian M. Bruel MD ▪ Susan Orillosa MD ▪ Karina Bouffard MD

Interventional Procedures for Cancer Pain

- One of the major components of cancer care is to treat the cancer-related pain that affects patients throughout their disease course, treatment, and recovery.
- Pain may present either from primary disease, cancer-related treatments, comorbid conditions, or an interaction among these etiologies.
- Cancer pain may manifest after surgery, radiation, chemotherapy, and immunotherapy.
- Cancer pain is typically nociceptive, visceral, neuropathic, or due to a combination of these.
- Interventional procedures have been used to help control the pain and are commonly used in conjunction with other modalities, such as oral medications and behavioral therapy. These techniques may also be more appropriate in patients who are unable to tolerate side effects of systemic medications. Some examples of interventional techniques for cancer related pain are listed here.

Intraspinal analgesia

Epidural

- The most common procedure for spinal or radicular pain caused by primary or metastatic lesions that may affect intervertebral disks, nerve roots, or spinal canal size.
- Can provide highly selective pain relief and results in regional analgesia
- Epidural injections can be performed at the cervical, thoracic, lumbar, or caudal levels.
- Can be performed as a single injection, usually delivering a mixture of a steroid with or without local anesthetics
- Can also be performed via a temporary catheter that allows for continuous infusion of opioids, local anesthetics, or other adjuvant medications

Neurolytic procedures

- Neurolytic procedures are useful in neuropathic and/or visceral pain in the distribution of specific peripheral sensory and visceral afferent nerves.

- Chemical and thermal neurolysis have been performed to help provide pain relief.
- Commonly performed following a diagnostic nerve block using local anesthetic

Chemical neurolysis

- Ethyl alcohol (98%–100%) or phenol (5%–10%)
- Procedural options include:
  - Hyperbaric phenol saddle block for midline perineal pain in patients with rectal and pelvic malignancies
  - Celiac plexus/splanchnic block for visceral pain of gastrointestinal origin, particularly common with patients with pancreatic cancer
  - Intrapleural phenol block for visceral pain associated with esophageal cancer
  - Superior hypogastric plexus block for tumor extension into the pelvis
  - Ganglion impar block for visceral pain of the perineum

Radiofrequency thermal ablation

- Thermal neurolysis of nerves is typically used for regional pain from tumor burden or the consequences of cancer treatments.
- Radiofrequency ablation of the Gasserian ganglion or terminal branches of the trigeminal nerve for cancer-related facial pain may be indicated for carefully selected patients.
- More frequently, paravertebral, intercostal, or peripheral sensory nerves are targets for thermal ablation.

Nerve blocks

- Target regional symptoms in the distribution of single or multiple peripheral nerves.
- Steroid with or without local anesthetic is injected and can provide pain relief.
- Provides short- and potentially long-term benefits; permanent pain relief is not expected.
- Common nerve blocks include, but are not limited to, the following:
  - Stellate ganglion block for upper extremity pain and complex regional pain syndrome

III: Cancer- or Treatment-Related Symptoms

101

– Lumbar sympathetic chain block for lower extremity pain and complex regional pain syndrome
– Paravertebral or intercostal nerve blocks for intercostal neuralgia commonly seen with postthoracotomy pain syndrome

Spinal cord stimulation

- Considered for chronic neuropathic pain, usually resulting from cancer-related treatments. Indications include chronic regional pain syndrome, refractory postherpetic neuralgia, chemotherapy-induced peripheral neuropathy, and postradiation and surgical nerve injury in the cancer population.
- Prior to permanent implantation, patients undergo a spinal cord stimulator trial for 3 to 7 days. Implantation of a permanent system is performed only after a successful trial and after psychological clearance.

Peripheral nerve stimulation

- Has the same indications as spinal stimulation; however, the utility is limited to neuropathic pain involving specific nondermatomal peripheral nerves.
- May be placed in the suboccipital region for migraine headaches.
- Provides an alternative to regional nerve blocks.

Intrathecal drug delivery system

- Targeted delivery of analgesics to spinal cord pain receptors via intrathecal delivery of the medications through a catheter
- Allows for reduction of side effects typically associated with higher dosages of systemic medications.
- Intrathecal trials are often performed via continuous infusion of analgesia or a single intrathecal injection.
- FDA-approved analgesics typically used include morphine and ziconotide.
- Other options for carefully selected patients include the following: hydromorphone, fentanyl, sufentanil, bupivacaine, clonidine, and baclofen.

Vertebral augmentation procedures

- Kyphoplasty or vertebroplasty can be performed for painful vertebral compression fractures. Most commonly performed for multiple myeloma and fractures related to spinal metastasis (breast, lung, and prostate cancers).
- Multiple levels can be performed at one time on carefully selected patients.
- Careful review of diagnostic imaging must take place prior to the procedure to ensure that the posterior vertebral cortex is intact and to ensure that the fracture is not planar or with very significant reduction of vertebral body height.

Neurosurgical procedures

With a multidisciplinary approach to pain management and with a wide array of pharmacologic treatments for pain, few patients require neurosurgical intervention to interrupt nociceptive pathways. However, in patients who have failed other treatments, neurosurgical procedures for pain management may be considered.

Cordotomy

- This is the most commonly performed neurosurgical procedure for cancer pain.
- The goal is ablation of the spinothalamic tract, performed on the side contralateral to the patient's pain.
- Selection criteria: unilateral, somatic nociceptive type pain that is below the neck
- Less helpful in neuropathic pain owing to central sensitization.
- Performed via a laminectomy approach or, more commonly, percutaneously under CT guidance using radiofrequency ablation.
- In a large study, pain relief was achieved in the cancer population in 83%, but more studies are needed to determine efficacy.

Trigeminal tractotomy–nucleotomy

- Ablation of the spinal trigeminal tract and the nucleus caudalis at the craniocervical junction
- Selection criteria: unilateral, craniofacial cancer pain
- Performed percutaneously under CT guidance using radiofrequency ablation on the ipsilateral side of the patient's pain.
- Has similar success rates to percutaneous cordotomy, but more studies are needed.

Myelotomy

- Indicated in midline or bilateral pelvic or abdominal cancer pain.
- Midline or commissural myelotomy seeks to interrupt the deccusating fibers of the spinothalamic tract as they cross in the anterior white commissure of the spinal cord.
- The spinal lesion is created over several spinal cord segments at the lower thoracic area and is performed using radiofrequency or microsurgical techniques.
- The overall efficacy of midline myelotomy has been reported to be about 70%, but this is a procedure that is infrequently performed and more studies are needed.

Dorsal root entry zone (DREZ) lesioning

- Indicated in the treatment of localized, segmental pain associated with peripheral nerve, root, or spinal cord lesions
- The dorsal root entry zone includes the central portion of the dorsal spinal rootlets, Lissauer's tract, and layers I to V of Rexed's lamina. DREZotomy seeks to selectively destroy these areas.
- For cancer pain, DREZotomy involves elevation of the dorsal rootlets to allow lesioning in the ventrolateral portion of the root entry zone.
- This can be performed via microsurgical, radiofrequency, ultrasonic, and laser ablation.
- Best studied in Pancoast tumor and radiation-induced plexopathy

Helpful Hints

- Multidisciplinary and oftentimes a multimodal approach incorporating well-selected interventional therapies may improve pain control in cancer patients.
- Interventional pain therapies include nerve blocks, implantable devices, vertebral augmentation, and neurodestructive procedures. When considering these therapies, referral to an interventional pain specialist is recommended.

Suggested Readings

Benzon H, Rathmell JP, Wu CL, et al. *Raj's Practical Management of Pain*. Philadelphia, PA: Elsevier; 2008.

Benzon HT, Raja S, Molloy RE, et al. *Essentials of Pain Medicine and Regional Anesthesia*. New York, NY: WB Saunders-Churchill Livingstone; 2005.

Burton AW, Fisch MJ. *Cancer Pain Management*. New York, NY: McGraw Hill Companies, Inc; 2007.

Christo PJ, Mazloomdoost D. Interventional pain treatments for cancer pain. *Ann NY Acad Sci*. 2008;1138:299–328.

Deer TR, Prager J, Levy R, et al. Polyanalgesic Consensus Conference 2012: Recommendations for the management of pain by intrathecal (intraspinal) drug delivery: Report of an interdisciplinary expert panel. *Neuromodulation*. 2012;15(5):436–464.

Fitzgibbon D, Loeser J. *Cancer Pain: Assessment, Diagnosis, and Management*. Philadelphia, PA: Lippincott Williams & Wilkins; 2010.

Gadgil N, Viswanathan A. DREZotomy in the treatment of cancer pain: A review. *Stereotact Funct Neurosurg*. 2012;90(6):356–360.

Kanpolat Y, Ugur HC, Ayten M, et al. Computed tomography guided percutaneous cordotomy for intractable pain in malignancy. *Neurosurgery*. 2009;64(3 suppl): 187–193.

Loeser JD, ed. *Bonica's Management of Pain* (3rd ed.). Philadelphia, PA: Lippincott Williams & Wilkins; 2001.

III: Cancer- or Treatment-Related Symptoms

Paraneoplastic Syndromes Affecting the Nervous System

Rajesh R. Yadav MD

Description

Paraneoplastic syndrome refers to signs and symptoms which can occur with organ or tissue damage from the nonmetastatic remote effects of cancer.

Paraneoplastic neurological disorders (PND) occur with damage to one or multiple areas involving tissues ranging from the cerebral cortex to the neuromuscular junction, nerves, and muscles. Examples include limbic encephalitis, cerebellar degeneration, neuropathy, neuromuscular junction pathologies such as Lambert–Eaton myasthenic syndrome (LEMS), and myasthenia gravis (MG).

Epidemiology

- Incidence varies based on the tumor type and neurologic syndrome.
- Lung cancers, especially small cell lung cancer, account for a disproportionate number and variety of PND.
- LEMS occurs in 3% of lung cancer patients.
- With thymoma, MG incidence rate may be 10% to 15%.
- Overall incidence appears to be low, with less than 1% of all cancer patients being affected.
- Plasma cell dyscrasia-related paraneoplastic peripheral neuropathy incidence rate is reported at 5% to 15%.
- With rare osteosclerotic forms of myeloma, there is a higher than 50% probability of developing a predominantly motor paraneoplastic peripheral neuropathy.

Pathogenesis

- These syndromes occur when antibodies are made against tumors that express nervous system proteins.
- Antibodies may be detectable in serum and cerebrospinal fluid (CSF) in many of the patients.
- Localized and multifocal immunological attacks produce a myriad of symptoms and functional deficits.

Clinical Features

- Paraneoplastic syndromes can produce persistent neurologic deficits and functional decline.
- The extent of the neurological involvement and severity dictates the functional impact.
- The treatment(s) and potential improvements must be considered when establishing rehabilitation goals.
- With significant encephalomyelitis and associated bulbar deficits, respiratory, communication, and nutritional issues may develop.

Diagnosis

- In the case of prior cancer history, PND should prompt workup for malignancy recurrence or progression.

Differential diagnosis

- Peripheral and autonomic neuropathies associated with chemotherapy
- Tumor recurrence
- Plexopathies
- Leptomeningeal disease with tumor progression
- Cognitive decline with medications and infections

History

- Many PNDs occur during earlier stages of cancer prior to cancer diagnosis.
- Symptoms such as weakness, sensory changes, ataxia, cognitive deficits, and autonomic dysfunction can develop and advance over days to weeks and then may plateau.

Signs and symptoms

- Limbic encephalitis:
  - Associated with testicular germ cell tumors
  - Cognitive deficits, including hallucinations, memory loss, and anxiety
- Encephalomyelitis:
  - Associated with small cell lung cancer, breast cancer, and thymoma
  - Cognitive, sensory, bulbar, and motor deficits
  - Ataxia
- Cerebellar degeneration:
  - Associated malignancies: small cell lung cancer, breast cancer, gynecological tumors, and Hodgkin's lymphoma
  - Limb and truncal ataxia

- Paraneoplastic opsoclonus–myoclonus ataxia:
  - Rare syndrome presents with brain stem dysfunction, imbalance, nausea, vomiting, or vertigo.
  - Ataxia and cerebellar tremor may be associated with opsoclonus "dancing eyes" and systemic myoclonus.
- Eye movements can include rapid and direction changing nystagmus, which is worsened with volitional eye movements.
- Symmetric or asymmetric ataxia is often severe, and limits ambulation and functional activities of daily living.
- There is a variable amount of ataxia, opsoclonus, and myoclonus.
  - Associated with breast, gynecologic, and bronchogenic carcinoma
- Subacute motor neuropathy:
  - Usually there is an underlying diagnosis of Hodgkin's or non-Hodgkin's lymphoma.
  - It is a motor neuron-only disease and there are generally no upper motor neuron signs.
  - Sensory loss is mild or absent.
  - There is a subacute, progressive, painless, bilateral, but slightly asymmetric weakness that starts in the lower extremities and may ultimately affect the upper extremities.
- Lambert–Eaton myasthenic syndrome:
  - Associated with small cell lung cancer
  - Symmetrical slowly progressive proximal muscle weakness, which improves temporarily with exercise
  - Areflexia, autonomic dysfunction, and cranial ocular symptoms may be present.

Testing
- Diagnostic workup can include brain MRI, positron emission tomography (PET) scan, serum and CSF studies.
- Brain MRI can assist with diagnosis of limbic encephalitis.
- Screening studies can direct one toward search of an occult malignancy.
  - Examples include P/Q type voltage-gated calcium channel antibodies, acetylcholine receptor antibodies, and anti-Hu antibodies associated with paraneoplastic encephalomyelitis.

Treatment
- Timely diagnosis and treatment of the tumor is of crucial importance in managing PND.

- Adjuvant treatments can include intravenous immunoglobulins, plasmapheresis, corticosteroids, and immunosuppressants.
- In general treatment of the paraneoplastic syndromes, except polymyositis, Lambert-Eaton myasthenic syndrome and opsoclonus-myoclonus syndrome has been relatively ineffective.
- Treament with corticosteroids, chemotherapeutic agents, plasmapheresis, and intravenous immunoglobulins have been unsuccessful.
- Occasional patients respond to tumor resection or systemic treatment.
- Treatments often are supportive.
- Opsoclonus–myoclonus syndrome is usually progressive, but may respond to corticosteroids or adrenocorticotropic hormone (ACTH).
- Lambert–Eaton myasthenic syndrome may respond to tumor removal or treatment, immunosuppression, intravenous immunoglobulin, and plasmapheresis.
- Many patients with dermatomyositis and polymyositis improve with immunosuppressive therapy.
- With subacute motor neuropathy, there may be spontaneous stabilization or improvement after a period of months or years, and this period is not reduced with anti-inflammatory treatment.

Prognosis
- Spontaneous improvement is rare, although symptoms may plateau.
- Depends on the underlying disease process and its response to the treatment.

Helpful Hints
- A variety of neurologic symptoms may occur and may be associated with malignancies.
- More obvious etiologies for neurological decline should first be ruled out.

Suggested Readings
Dalmau JD, Rosenfeld MR. Overview of paraneoplastic syndromes of the nervous system. *UpToDate*, 2011.
Darnell RB, Posner JB. Paraneoplastic syndromes affecting the nervous system. *Semin Oncol.* 2006;33:270–298.
Levin VA. *Cancer in the Nervous System.* 2nd ed. New York, NY: Oxford University Press; 2002:423–437.
Rees J. Paraneoplastic syndromes. *Curr Opin Neurol.* 1998;11(6):633–637.

III: Cancer- or Treatment-Related Symptoms

Plexopathy: Brachial

Ying Guo MD MS

Description
Dysfunction of the peripheral nerve network that originates from the cervical and upper thoracic nerve roots and terminates at the upper extremity nerves.

Etiology/Types
- Direct pressure by a tumor mass
- Invasion of nerve by cancer cells
- Radiation can cause direct injury to the axons, indirect injury to small intraneural tissues, or ischemic changes to axons with multifocal denervation.
- Head and neck or thoracic surgery with traction of the brachial plexus can lead to nerve damage. Also caused by head and neck- or pulmonary-based tumor compression or invasion.
- Idiopathic brachial plexopathy can also occur postoperatively; felt to be an inflammatory disorder.

Epidemiology
- Cancer-related brachial plexopathy: 0.4% (most frequent cancers are breast and lung cancer)
- Radiation-related brachial plexopathy: 2% to 5%
- Idiopathic brachial plexopathy (also known as Parsonage–Turner syndrome, paralytic brachial neuritis, brachial plexus neuropathy, acute brachial radiculitis, or brachial amyotrophy) has an estimated annual incidence of 2 to 3 per 100,000.

Pathogenesis
- Most related to axonal loss
- Demyelination
- Combination of both

Clinical Features
- Decreased sensation and strength in the upper extremity lead to impairment of activities of daily living. Pain can cause further limitation in function.

Diagnosis

History
- Chronic progression of symptoms in patients with a history of cancer (breast and lung cancer) and radiation treatment suggest either as a cause.

- More acute onset is associated with idiopathic brachial plexopathy or traction injury.

Examination
- A Horner syndrome in the setting of shoulder pain and weakness is strongly suggestive of a pulmonary tumor.
- Sensory loss
- Pain
- Weakness and atrophy
- Tendon reflexes may be reduced in weak muscles.

Testing
- Nerve conduction and electromyography (EMG): Sensory deficits are found in the distribution of dermatome (C5-lateral antebrachial nerve, C6-radial nerve, C7-median nerve at middle finger, C8-ulnar nerve, T1-medial antebrachial nerve). Motor nerve conduction study of all three nerves (radial, ulnar, and median) should be assessed; EMG of muscles; at least two muscles per peripheral nerve, and two muscles of each myotome should be tested. Abnormal spontaneous activity in the muscle may not appear until 3 weeks after the acute onset of plexopathies. Myokymic discharges can be seen in radiation-induced plexopathy.
- MRI: Magnetic resonance neurography is a specialized procedure that can visualize individual roots, segments of the plexus, and peripheral nerves and can be used to assess surgically remediable lesions.

Differential diagnosis
- Differentiate cancer recurrence versus radiation plexopathy (Table 45.1)
- Thoracic outlet syndrome

Treatment
- Cancer: radiation, chemotherapy; treat neuropathic pain with gabapentin, pregabalin; surgery; can be associated with lymphedema
- Radiation-induced brachial plexopathy: symptom management, maintain range of motion

Table 45.1　Differentiating Plexopathy Due to Tumor Versus Radiation

	Tumor	Radiation
Pain at onset	+++	+
Paresthesia	+	+++
Weakness	+	++
EMG		Fasciculations Myokymic discharges
Location	Lower plexus (inferior trunk and medial cord)	Upper plexus

+ Weak association.

+++ Strong association.

Helpful Hints

- When a cancer patient develops weakness or numbness, always put cancer in the differential diagnosis.
- Inform oncologist when patient presents with new onset of brachial plexopathy.
- Correct diagnosis can help the patient cope with his or her disability.

Suggested Readings

Johansson S, Svensson H, Denekamp J. Dose response and latency for radiation-induced fibrosis, edema, and neuropathy in breast cancer patients. *Int J Radiat Oncol Biol Phys.* 2002;52(5):1207.

Kori SH. Diagnosis and management of brachial plexus lesions in cancer patients. *Oncology.* 1995;9(8):756–765.

Plexopathy: Lumbosacral

Ying Guo MD MS

Description

Dysfunction of the peripheral nerve network that originates from the lumbar and sacral nerve roots and terminates as the lower extremity nerves that innervate the muscles and skin of the legs and feet.

Etiology/Types

- Tumor related: primary or metastatic cancer invasion or compression of the plexus (caused by colorectal, breast, lung, gastric, thyroid, renal, ureteral, bladder, testicular, penile, prostate, cervical, ovarian, uterine, vaginal cancers, melanoma, lymphoma, schwannoma, chordoma, sarcoma, neurofibromas)
- Radiation plexopathy
- Retroperitoneal hematoma (anticoagulation)
- Abscess: patient usually has a history of abdominal or pelvic surgery.

Epidemiology

The incidence of lumbar plexopathy is unknown.

Pathogenesis

- Most related to axonal loss
- Radiation plexopathy is caused by tissue fibrosis, axonal injury by radiation, and microinfarction.

Clinical Features

- Decreased sensation and strength in the lower extremity lead to impairment of transfers and ambulation.
- Pain can cause further limitations in function and quality of life.

Diagnosis

Differential diagnosis

- Cancer recurrence versus radiation plexopathy (Table 46.1).

- Lumbosacral radiculopathy: paraspinal electromyogram (EMG) and sensory nerve conduction studies can help differentiate.
- Cauda equina syndrome: patient presents with neurogenic bladder and bowel symptoms and may have decreased rectal sensation and tone.
- Retroperitoneal hemorrhage or iliopsoas hematoma: acute onset, decrease in hemoglobin, and ecchymoses

History

- Chronic progression of symptoms in patients with a history of cancer and radiation treatment can suggest either as a cause.
- Acute onset can be associated with hematoma.
- Subacute onset is seen in abscess-induced lumbosacral plexopathy. A history of radiation to the abdominal/pelvic area and history of surgery should raise the alert for possible visceral perforation.

Examination

- Detailed assessment of bilateral lower extremity motor strength, sensation, and deep tendon reflexes
- Palpation of the inguinal region for possible hematoma

Testing

- Nerve conduction and EMG: Sensory nerve conduction studies: sural, superficial peroneal, medial plantar, and saphenous sensory nerves. Motor nerve conduction studies: femoral, tibial, and peroneal nerves. H-waves. EMG of muscles: at least two muscles per peripheral nerve, two muscles of each myotome and the paraspinal muscles on each level should be sampled.
  - Abnormal spontaneous activity in the muscle may not appear until 3 weeks after the acute onset of plexopathies.

Table 46.1   Differentiating Tumor From Radiation-Induced Lumbar Plexopathy

	Tumor	Radiation
Pain	can be severe early, can radiate	mild
Paresthesia	later	
Weakness	later	early
Location	lower plexus	upper plexus

– Upper limb nerve conduction study (NCS) should be performed to exclude polyneuropathy if symptoms are bilateral or diffuse.
– Myokymic motor units can be seen with radiation involvement.
■ CT and MRI: can help rule out cancer recurrence, hematoma, or abscess

Treatment

■ Cancer: radiation, chemotherapy, pharmacological management, and surgery
■ For patients with neuropathic pain: gabapentin, pregabalin, duloxetine, amitriptyline, or venlafaxine may be used for symptom management.
■ Radiation-induced brachial plexopathy: symptom management and physical and occupational therapy to increase function

Prognosis

■ Prognosis of plexopathy caused by recurrent cancer depends on cancer treatment.

■ Plexopathy caused by radiation usually has a slowly progressive course.
■ Plexopathy caused by hematoma has a relatively good prognosis for functional recovery.

Helpful Hints

■ Apply rehabilitation principles according to the patient's sensation loss and weakness.
■ Finding out the etiology can help patients to cope with their disability.

Suggested Readings

Jaeckle KA, Young DF, Foley KM. The natural history of lumbosacral plexopathy in cancer. *Neurology.* 1985;35(1):8–15.

Ladha SS, Spinner RJ, Suarez GA, et al. Neoplastic lumbosacral radiculoplexopathy in prostate cancer by direct perineural spread: An unusual entity. *Muscle Nerve.* 2006;34(5):659–665.

Planner AC, Donaghy M, Moore NR. Causes of lumbosacral plexopathy. *Clin Radiol.* 2006;61(12):987–995.

Thomas JE, Cascino TL, Earle JD. Differential diagnosis between radiation and tumor plexopathy of the pelvis. *Neurology.* 1985;35(1):1–7.

III: Cancer- or Treatment-Related Symptoms

Pressure Ulcers

Cynthia A. Worley BSN RN CWOCN

Description

The National Pressure Ulcer Advisory Panel (NPUAP) defines a pressure ulcer as an area of localized injury to the skin and/or underlying tissue usually over a bony prominence, as a result of pressure, or pressure in combination with shear.

Etiology

- Excessive pressure results in ischemia and necrosis.
- There is an inverse relationship between duration of pressure and amount of pressure needed. Low amounts of pressure over long periods of time can cause as much damage as high amounts of pressure for a short duration.
- Some body tissues are better able to withstand pressure than other areas (i.e., muscle is more sensitive to pressure than skin).
- Both intrinsic and extrinsic factors play a role in the development of pressure ulcers.

Epidemiology

- Incidence of pressure ulcers in an acute care setting is 7% to 9%, long-term care incidence is estimated to be between 3% and 31%, home care estimates incidence at 0% to 17%.
- Prevalence of pressure ulcers within the acute care setting is estimated to be between 14% and 17%, long-term care is 27%, and home care prevalence is estimated to range from 3% to 10%.
- Pressure ulcers most often occur in persons with advanced illnesses in acute and long-term care settings.

Pathogenesis

- Deep tissue injury occurs first from a V-shaped pressure gradient. The gradient results when the upward force from a supporting surface is exerted against a downward force exerted by the bony prominence.
- Pressure is greatest at the apex of the gradient and lessens to the sides as it approaches the surface. The tip of the "V" is at its deepest point.
- Blood vessels, subcutaneous fat, fascia, and muscle are compressed between the two forces.

- Shearing injuries result when mechanical force is exerted parallel to a tissue area. The bone and attached structures slide under the skin while the skin remains relatively stationary and held in place by friction between the skin and the supporting surface. The sliding causes compression of blood vessels and ischemia.

Risk Factors

- Impaired sensory perception
- Moisture
- Decreased activity
- Impaired mobility
- Decreased nutrition
- Friction/shear forces
- Advanced age
- Male gender
- African American race
- Low body mass index
- Urinary or fecal incontinence
- Use of restraints
- Fever/sepsis
- Hypotension
- Dehydration
- Anemia
- Immunosuppression
- Renal failure
- Comorbidities such as diabetes and malignancy
- Cachexia
- Fatigue is responsible for lower activity levels and muscle wasting.
- Protein degradation contributes to a compromised immune status and decreases survival rates.

Clinical Features

- The NPUAP has developed a staging system for pressure ulcers. Stages are I to IV, suspected deep tissue injury, and unstageable.
- Determination of stage is dependent on visualization and identification of the deepest layer of viable tissue. No patient's ulcer should be staged if covered with nonviable tissue.
- Stage I is described as "intact skin with nonblanchable redness of a localized area, usually over a bony

prominence. Darkly pigmented skin may not have visible blanching; its color may differ from the surrounding area."

- Stage II is described as "partial thickness loss of dermis presenting as a shallow open ulcer with a red pink wound bed, without slough. May also present as an intact or open/ruptured serum-filled blister."
- Stage III is described as "full thickness tissue loss. Subcutaneous fat may be visible but bone, tendon or muscle is not exposed. Slough may be present but does not obscure the depth of tissue loss. May include undermining and tunneling."
- Stage IV is described as "full-thickness tissue loss with exposed bone, tendon, or muscle. Slough or eschar may be present on some parts of the wound bed. Often includes undermining and tunneling."
- Suspected deep tissue injury is described as a "purple or maroon localized area of discolored intact skin or blood-filled blister due to damage of underlying soft tissue from pressure and/or shear."
- "Unstageable" is used to describe a "full thickness tissue loss in which the base of the ulcer is covered by slough (yellow, tan, gray, green, or brown) and/or eschar (tan, brown, or black) in the wound bed."

Natural History
- An area of nonblanchable erythema may or may not evolve into a greater area of tissue destruction.
- Superficial ulcers heal by regeneration, as the destroyed tissue is replaced with the same tissue type.
- Full-thickness ulcers heal by repair as the destroyed tissue cannot be replaced. The defect is filled with scar tissue.
- Urinary and/or fecal incontinence can play a significant role in pressure ulcer development.
- There is a strong linear correlation between pressure ulcer risk and performance status in patients with advanced illness.

Diagnosis
- History, physical examination, and risk factor assessment
- Current cancer treatment, including last chemotherapy course and radiation treatment
- Test red areas over bony prominences by gently pressing on the area; if the area blanches, this is not a pressure-related injury.
- The Braden Scale (Table 47.1) is the most widely used risk assessment tool for pressure ulcers in the

United States. It consists of six subscales containing a numerical range of scores. The lower the cumulative score, the greater the risk for development of pressure ulcers.

Treatment
Medical
- Off-loading pressure through use of a turning schedule if the patient cannot get out of bed
- Frequent position changes for the wheelchair user
- Use of appropriate support surfaces both for the bed and wheelchair
- Weekly Braden risk assessment following an initial baseline score
- Nutritional consultation if Braden score is low
- Physical therapy consult for mobility issues
- Address incontinence issues
- Routine scrutiny of appropriate lab values as they relate to wound healing and appropriate interventions as needed

Surgical
- Sharp debridement of devitalized tissue if allowed by patient's immune status.
- Plastic surgery, including flap coverage

Topical dressings
- Assessment of wound characteristics and determination of appropriate topical dressings:
  - Scant or small amounts of drainage—foam dressing, hydrocolloid, gel/gauze dressing, composite. dressing, transparent film
  - Moderate drainage—foam dressing, calcium alginate, or hydrofiber
    - Deeper wounds will require a "filler" dressing and a cover dressing.
  - High or large amounts of drainage—consider a negative pressure drainage management system, calcium alginate/foam dressing combination, and increase the frequency of dressing changes.

Prognosis
- Healing is dependent on the patient and the medical condition.
- The healed ulcer area has decreased tissue tolerance and will be at risk for reinjury without proper prevention measures.
- The patient should be monitored throughout the cancer treatment and observed for signs of wound degradation.

Table 47.1 Braden Scale for Predicting Pressure-Sore Risk

Patient's Name _____ Evaluator's Name _____ Date of Assessment _____

	1	2	3	4			
SENSORY PERCEPTION ability to respond meaningfully to pressure-related discomfort	**1. Completely Limited** Unresponsive (does not mean, finch, or grasp) to painful stimuli, due to diminished level of consciousness or sedation, OR limited ability to feel pain over most of body.	**2. Very Limited** Responds only to painful stimuli. Cannot communicate discomfort except by moaning or restlessness OR has a sensory impairment that limits the ability to feel pain or discomfort over 50% of body.	**3. Slightly Limited** Responds to verbal commands, but cannot always communicate discomfort or the need to be turned OR has some sensory impairment that limits ability to feel pain or discomfort in one or two extremities.	**4. No Impairment** Responds to verbal commands. Has no sensory deficit that would limit ability to feel or voice pain or discomfort.			
MOISTURE degree to which skin is exposed to moisture	**1. Constantly Moist** Skin is kept moist almost constantly by perspiration, urine, etc. Dampness is detected every time patient is moved or turned.	**2. Very Moist** Skin is often, but not always moist. Linen must be changed at least once a shift.	**3. Occasionally Moist** Skin is occasionally moist, requiring an extra linen change approximately once a day.	**4. Rarely Moist** Skin is usually dry, linen only requires changing at routine intervals.			
ACTIVITY degree of physical activity	**1. Bedfast** Confined to bed.	**2. Chairfast** Ability to walk severely limited or non-existent. Cannot bear own weight and/or must be assisted into chair or wheelchair.	**3. Walks Occasionally** Walks occasionally during day, but for very short distances, with or without assistance. Spends majority of each shift in bed or chair.	**4. Walks Frequently** Walks outside room at least twice a day and inside room at least once every 2 hours during waking hours.			
MOBILITY ability to change and control body position	**1. Completely Immobile** Does not make even slight changes in body or extremity position without assistance.	**2. Very Limited** Make occasional slight changes in body or extremity position but unable to make frequent or significant changes independently.	**3. Slightly Limited** Makes frequent though slight changes in body or extremity position independently.	**4. No Limitation** Makes major and frequent changes in position without assistance.			
NUTRITION usual food intake pattern	**1. Very Poor** Never eats a complete meal. Rarely eats more than 33% of any food offered. Eats two servings or less of protein (meat or dairy products) per day. Takes fluids poorly. Does not take a liquid dietary supplement OR is NPO (nothing per os) and/or maintained on clear liquids or IVs for more than 5 days.	**2. Probably Inadequate** Rarely eats a complete meal and generally eats only about 50% of any food offered. Protein intake includes only three servings of meat or dairy products per day. Occasionally will take a dietary supplement OR receives less than optimum amount of liquid diet or tube feeding.	**3. Adequate** Eats over half of most meals. Eats a total of four servings of protein (meat, dairy products per day). Occasionally will refuse a meal, but will usually take a supplement when offered OR is on a tube feeding or TPN (total parenteral nutrition) regimen, which probably meets most of nutritional needs.	**4. Excellent** Eats most of every meal. Never refuses a meal. Usually eats a total of four or more servings of meat and dairy products. Occasionally eats between meals. Does not require supplementation.			
FRICTION & SHEAR	**1. Problem** Requires moderate to maximum assistance in moving. Complete lifting without sliding against sheets is impossible. Frequently slides down in bed or chair, requiring frequent repositioning with maximum assistance. Spasticity, contractures, or agitation leads to almost constant friction.	**2. Potential Problem** Moves feebly or requires minimum assistance. During a move skin probably slides to some extent against sheets, chair, restraints or other devices. Maintains relatively good position in chair or bed most of the time but occasionally slides down.	**3. No Apparent Problem** Moves in bed and in chair independently and has sufficient muscle strength to lift up completely during move. Maintains good position in bed or chair.				
							Total Score

112

Helpful Hints

- Observe for signs and symptoms of infection and treat both systemically and topically as appropriate.
- Change topical therapy as the wound conditions change.
- If no improvement within 2-week time frame, complete reassessment may be necessary to determine failure to improve.

Suggested Readings

Lyder C. Assessing risk and preventing pressure ulcers in patients with cancer. *Semin Oncol Nurs.* 2006;22(3):178–184.

Maida V, Corbo M, Dolzhykov M, et al. Wounds in advanced illness: A prevalence and incidence study based on a prospective case series. *Int Wound J.* 2008;5(2):305–314.

Maida V, Lau F, Downing M, et al. Correlation between Braden Scald and Palliative Performance Scale in advanced illness. *Int Wound J.* 2008;5(4)585–590.

National Pressure Ulcer Advisory Panel. http://www.npuap.org

III: Cancer- or Treatment-Related Symptoms

Pulmonary: Pleural Effusions

Carlos A. Jimenez MD

Description
Pleural effusions in cancer patients have significant therapeutic and prognostic implications, whether or not malignant cells are identified in the fluid. Because malignant pleural effusions often signal advanced disease and incurability, treatment alternatives are frequently directed toward palliation.

Etiology
- Almost any type of cancer can affect the pleural cavity.
- Lung cancer accounts for up to half of the malignant pleural effusions, followed in frequency by breast cancer.
- 17% of the pleural effusions in cancer patients are "paramalignant," as they are not caused by direct malignant involvement of the pleural cavity, but as a result of local or systemic effects of the tumor, complications of cancer therapy, or concurrent nonmalignant disease.

Epidemiology
- The estimated incidence of malignant pleural effusions in the United States is 150,000 cases annually.

Pathogenesis
- In addition to direct tumor involvement of the pleura, malignant pleural effusions can occur from lymphatic blockage and elevated local production of vascular endothelial growth factor (VEGF).
- Lymphatic obstruction is the most common cause of paramalignant effusions.
- Other causes of paramalignant effusions are:
  - Bronchial obstruction
  - Nonreexpandable lung
  - Pulmonary embolism
  - Pneumonia

Risk Factors
- Metastatic disease
- Malignant mediastinal lymphadenopathy
- Pneumonia
- Congestive heart failure

Clinical Features
Patients can present with shortness of breath (dyspnea), cough, or chest pain.

Diagnosis

Differential diagnosis
- Analysis of pleural fluid is paramount to determine its cause.
- The differential diagnosis of pleural effusion is extensive and can include parapneumonic process, neoplasm, pulmonary embolism, rheumatoid arthritis, pancreatitis, post myocardial infarction (MI), and autoimmune disease.

History
- Gradual onset of dyspnea on exertion
- Cough may occur with large effusions.

Examination
- Dullness on percussion of the affected hemithorax
- Absence of breathing sounds on auscultation of the affected hemithorax.

Testing
- Pleural fluid cytology reveals malignant cells in approximately two thirds of malignant pleural effusions.
- Pleural biopsies might be indicated in certain situations when the cause of pleural fluid is uncertain or to confirm malignant involvement of the pleural cavity.

Functional impact
- Worsening performance status may impact the patient's ability to receive further treatment for cancer.
- Undrained moderate or large size parapneumonic effusions might impair response to antibiotic treatment.

Treatment
- Treatment is directed toward the cause of pleural effusion.
- Palliation of symptoms is tailored to individual patient needs.
- Important components of the evaluation to recommend the best palliative approach include:
  - Patient's preferences
  - Performance status and information regarding prior thoracenteses, including the volume of fluid

removed, whether lung reexpansion and palliation of dyspnea were achieved, and the time interval between repeated taps.

■ Oxygen therapy, opioids, repeated thoracentesis, indwelling pleural catheters, and pleurodesis are the most common alternatives to accomplish palliation.

Prognosis

■ Prognosis will be determined by the cause of the pleural effusion.

■ Patients with malignant pleural effusion, good performance status, and good lung reexpansion after a therapeutic thoracentesis have better results with palliative interventions and better tolerance to physical activity.

■ Deterioration of functional status as malignant disease progresses is expected.

Helpful Hints

■ Cancer patients presenting with a pleural effusion require a thorough evaluation to establish the etiology of pleural fluid accumulation in order to recommend the best treatment and palliative alternatives.

■ Use of an indwelling pleural catheter for regular drainage of a persistent pleural effusion can help some patients with advanced cancer tolerate more physical activity for a longer period of time.

Suggested Readings

Light RW, Lee YCG. *Textbook of Pleural Diseases*. London, UK: Hodder Arnold; 2008.

Uzbeck MH, Almeida FA, Sarkiss MG, et al. Management of malignant pleural effusions. *Adv Ther*. 2010;27(6): 334–347.

III: Cancer- or Treatment-Related Symptoms

Radiation Effects: Central Nervous System

Jack B. Fu MD

Description

Central nervous system (CNS) effects due to prior radiation treatment can include neurologic weakness and cognitive dysfunction.

Etiology/Types

- Acute reaction—within the first several weeks
- Early-delayed reaction—within 1 to 6 months of treatment
- Late-delayed reaction—months to years after treatment. This includes radiation necrosis

Epidemiology

- Radiation directed at the CNS is commonly performed for neoplastic lesions. Acute reaction effects are common.
- The risk of radiation late effects increases with higher overall doses, especially over 50 Gy.
- Radiation necrosis has been reported as often as 2% to 50% of patients receiving 30 Gy.

Pathogenesis

- Radiation is toxic to tumor cells. Despite efforts to focus the radiation on the lesion only, some collateral damage to neighboring cells is possible.
- Increased capillary permeability results in extracellular edema, demyelination, and coagulative necrosis.
- Also, there is evidence that neuroprogenitor cell activity is reduced.
- Vascular damage may result in recurrent ischemic cerebrovascular accidents.
- Vascular insults can be worsened with concomitant chemotherapy.

Risk Factors for Radiation Late Effects

- Age (less than 7 or more than 60)
- More than 2 Gy dose per fraction
- Higher cumulative dose
- Greater volume of brain irradiated
- Hyperfractionation schedules
- Shorter overall treatment time
- Concomitant or subsequent use of chemotherapy
- Presence of comorbid vascular risk factors

Clinical Features

- Cognitive changes/mental fatigue
- Seizures
- Headaches
- Upper motor neuron signs
- Weakness
- Numbness
- Ataxia and incoordination

Natural History

- Acute reaction—acute decline with focal deficits
- Early-delayed reaction—somnolence, fatigue, cognitive dysfunction
- Late-delayed reaction—usually irreversible and progressive, with deficits in memory, visual motor processing, quantitative skills, and attention months to years after.

Diagnosis

Differential diagnosis

- New metastatic CNS lesion
- Primary CNS lesion progression
- Seizures
- Cerebrovascular accident
- Brain abscess

History

- Progressive onset of weakness/incoordination
- Sensory changes
- Headache
- New cognitive changes
- Worsening or new onset seizure
- Falls
- Visual changes
- Worsening or new bowel dysfunction
- Worsening or new bladder dysfunction

Examination

- Sensory deficits
- Motor deficits/hemiparesis
- Cognitive deficits
- Dysphagia
- Aphasia

- Hyperreflexia/hypertonia
- Cranial nerve palsies
- Visual deficits

Testing
- MRI
- CT
- Neuropsychologic testing
- EEG (electroencephalogram) if suspect seizures
- Lumbar puncture may help evaluate for leptomeningeal disease.

Pitfalls
- Pathology may be indicated to better identify whether a lesion is recurrence versus radiation necrosis. However, often, radiology imaging is sufficient to determine this.

Treatment

Medical
- Medical treatment options are not well studied. However, some evidence suggests a benefit, although with limited success. Medical treatments can include:
  - Steroids
  - High-dose vitamins such as Vitamin E_1 (Alpha-tocopherol), Accutane (Isotretinoin)
  - Hyperbaric oxygen
  - Antiplatelet agents (e.g., aspirin)
  - Anticoagulants (e.g., low-molecular-weight heparin)
  - Tamoxifen
  - Bevacizumab
  - Pentoxifylline

Surgical
- Surgical resection of necrotic tissue is uncommon.
- It can be performed in patients who require removal owing to mass effect and hydrocephalus.

Exercises
- Exercises and therapy should address the neurologic deficits.
- Range-of-motion exercises for paralyzed limbs
- Training in activities of daily living, ambulation, transfers, and wheelchair mobility

Consults
- Physical medicine and rehabilitation
- Neurosurgery
- Neurooncology
- Neuropsychology
- Radiation oncology

Complications of treatment
- Surgical resection is rare and can result in worsening or new neurologic symptoms.
- Side effects for various medical treatments can occur, depending on the selected agent. Steroids are the most commonly used and can result in hyperglycemia, weight gain, and swelling.

Prognosis
- In acute and early-delayed, the prognosis is good.
- Neurological and functional recovery for radiation late effects/radiation necrosis is poor. Many patients suffer permanent neurologic symptoms. Nevertheless, efforts to recover lost function should be performed.

Helpful Hints
- Radiation late effects are difficult to treat and can be a frustrating condition to treat for both patient and clinician. Pharmacologic treatments have not been well studied and are not very effective. Neurologic recovery is usually limited.
- Often presents as a new neurologic deficit. The differential diagnosis can include tumor recurrence, seizures, cerebrovascular accident, and so forth. Workup includes imaging and may include biopsy if imaging is unable to identify the etiology.

Suggested Readings
Dietrich J, Monje M, Wefel J, Meyers C. Clinical patterns and biological correlates of cognitive dysfunction associated with cancer therapy. *Oncologist.* 2008;13:1285–1295.

Roman DD, Sperduto PW. Neuropsychological effects of cranial radiation: Current knowledge and future directions. *Int J Radiat Oncol Biol B.* 1995;31:983–998.

Sheline GE. Radiation therapy of brain tumors. *Cancer.* 1977;39:873–881.

III: Cancer- or Treatment-Related Symptoms

Radiation Effects: Myelitis

Rajesh R. Yadav MD

Description

Radiation myelitis is a form of spinal cord injury that may follow radiation treatment to the spine or surrounding region.

Etiology/Types

- Can be classified as:
  - Acute (early or transient)
  - Delayed

Epidemiology

- Since the initial description of postradiation spinal cord injury in the 1940s, technological advancements have limited the amount of undesired radiation to surrounding tissue(s).
- Myelopathy has been described in 5% of patients who survive 18 months after receiving 5,000 cGy for lung cancer.
- Incidence for transient radiation myelitis following mantle field irradiation for Hodgkin's disease is reported to be 10% to 15%.

Pathogenesis

- Spinal cord tolerance to radiation is dependent on cumulative dose and fraction size.
- White matter changes include:
  - Demyelination
  - Axonal loss
  - Focal necrosis
- Vascular changes consist of:
  - Telangiectasis
  - Endothelial swelling with fibrin exudation
  - Hyaline degeneration and thickening
  - Perivascular fibrosis
  - Vasculitis
  - Fibrinoid necrosis
- The transient nature of acute radiation injury is due to:
  - Axonal edema
  - Vascular necrosis
  - Diffuse transient demyelination
- Delayed late-radiation injury is more permanent and is felt to be due to intramedullary infarction or bleeding with vascular damage.

Risk Factors

- Radiation to the mantle field and spine
- Risk is dose related and more frequently seen with total radiation dose greater than 5,000 cGy or daily radiation fraction greater than 200 cGy.

Clinical Features

- Symptoms usually begin insidiously.
- Paresis, numbness, and sphincter dysfunction may be noted.
- Altered sensation can include decreased temperature or proprioception.
- Lower extremity weakness, foot drop, or complete paresis below the irradiation field
- Neurogenic bowel and bladder

Diagnosis

Differential diagnosis

- Tumor recurrence
- Spinal cord compression
- Spinal instability
- Plexopathy
- Peripheral neuropathy
- Leptomeningeal disease
- Trauma
- Vitamin B_{12} deficiency
- Paraneoplastic syndromes
- Demyelinating diseases, including multiple sclerosis

History

- Acute radiation injury:
  - Occurs weeks to months after completion of radiation treatment
  - Presents as intermittent, short-lived sensations described as symmetrical tingling, numbness, or electric shock extending from the neck to the limbs.
- Delayed radiation injury:
  - Often occurs 6 to 24 months after completion of radiation treatment but may be delayed by years
  - Shorter latency period is associated with higher radiation doses, larger doses per fraction, and childhood irradiation.

– Patients may have progressive neurologic decline and may have paraplegia or tetraplegia.
– Symptoms may be mild or severe.
– Functional deficits include sensory and motor abnormalities, bowel and bladder dysfunction, and diaphragmatic disturbance with high lesions.
– Brown-Sequard hemicord pattern begins more caudally and ascends to the irradiated level of cord.
– The neurologic deficits generally progress over several weeks to months and then plateau.
– Lower motor neuron syndrome may be present with radiation to lower spine and presents with radicular symptoms including slowly progressive lower extremity weakness and almost normal bladder and bowel function.
  • Patients may remain ambulatory for years despite increase in weakness.
■ Pain is usually not a prominent complaint.

Examination
■ Lhermitte's sign:
– Shocklike sensations from the neck to the extremities, typically brought on by neck flexion
– Occurs in a small number of patients (less than 4%) with median onset of 3 months and median duration of 6 months
■ Sensory deficits and motor weakness
■ Gait abnormality
■ Bowel and bladder dysfunction

Testing
■ Neuroimaging findings
– Low signal intensity on T1-weighted and high signal intensity on T2-weighted images along with variable edema
– May also be nonspecific
■ MRI is helpful in excluding other causes of myelopathy, including tumor.

Treatment
■ High-dose corticosteroids:
– Sometimes this treatment can lead to dramatic clinical and radiologic resolution.
■ Bevacizumab was used with success in a recent case study with delayed radiation injury and paraplegia.
■ There are a variety of other treatments that have had limited effectiveness.
■ Rehabilitation interventions should be prescribed for functional deficits including self-care activities of daily living, mobility, adaptive equipment, and family training.

Prognosis
■ Acute radiation injury symptoms often resolve spontaneously 2 to 9 months after onset.
■ Delayed myelopathy is permanent and the signs and symptoms rarely, if ever, resolve.

Helpful Hint
■ Radiation myelopathy should be in the differential diagnosis of patients with neurologic compromise and a history of radiation within the fields of the affected spine.

Suggested Readings
Chamberlain MC, Eaton KD, Fink J. Radiation-induced myelopathy: Treatment with bevacizumab. *Arch Neurol.* 2011;68(12):1608–1609.
Dropcho EJ. Central nervous system injury by therapeutic irradiation. *Neurol Clin.* 1991;9:969–988.
Gibbs IC, Patil C, Gerszten PC, et al. Delayed radiation-induced myelopathy after spinal radiosurgery. *Neurosurgery.* 2009;64(2):A67–A72.
Kavanaugh B. Complications of Spinal Irradiation. http://www.uptodate.com/contents/complications-of-spinal-cord-irradiation. Accessed April 12, 2013.
Mul VE, de Jong JM, Murrer LH, et al. Lhermitte sign and myelopathy after irradiation of the cervical spinal cord in radiotherapy treatment of head and neck cancer. *Strahlenther Onkol,* 2012;188(1):71–76.
Patchell RA, Posner JB. Neurologic complications of systemic cancer. *Neurol Clin.* 1985;3:729–750.
Rampling R, Symonds P. Radiation myelopathy. *Curr Opin Neurol.* 1998;11(6):627–632.

III: Cancer- or Treatment-Related Symptoms

Sacrectomy

Rajesh R. Yadav MD

Description

Total or partial sacral amputation is a technically challenging and rare procedure used to treat aggressive types of tumors.

Etiology

- Sacrectomy is performed for tumors, including:
  - Chordoma
  - Colorectal cancers
  - Giant cell tumors
  - Sarcomas
  - Neuroblastoma
  - Ganglioma
  - Schwannoma
  - Desmoid tumors
- Locally invasive tumors, such as rectal cancer, may also be treated in this manner.

Epidemiology

- Chordomas account for 36% of tumors leading to sacrectomy.
- Colorectal tumors—24%
- Sarcoma—22%
- Giant cell tumors—6%
- Others (neuroblastoma, ganglioma, schwanomma, and desmoid tumors)—12%

Pathogenesis

- Tumors may progress slowly over a period of months, leading to increasing symptoms.
- Depending on the extent of the tumor, patients may need sacrectomy via only posterior approach or both anterior and posterior approach.
  - Most nonrectal cancer—posterior approach only.
- In addition to the bony resection, neurolysis or nerve sacrifice may be necessary, depending on the extent of tumor involvement.
- Large skin defects following such a surgery often necessitate flap procedures, including myocutaneous flaps.

Risk Factors

- Unknown risk factors for most of the tumors.

Clinical Features

- Hip range of motion restrictions:
  - Flexion in particular is restricted significantly so as to not stretch the flap and impair healing.
- Restrictions with laying supine and sitting:
  - Often, patients have to lay in a side lying position.
  - Specific weight-bearing restrictions limiting sitting can continue for weeks.
    - Gradual easing of these restrictions is the norm.
    - Initial sitting may only be allowed with transfers.
- Altered weight bearing:
  - Depending on the flap used for reconstruction, altered weight bearing may follow.
- Multiple drains:
  - Drain management when performing activity.
- Significant wound care:
  - Close coordination of care with plastic surgery and the nursing staff is needed with any dressing changes and changes in functional restrictions due to wound-related concerns.
- Neurogenic bowel and bladder (lower motor neuron):
  - Especially with bilateral sacral nerve root ligation
- Significant pain
- Orthostatic symptoms

Diagnosis

Differential diagnosis

- Presence of low-back pain could be due to local mechanical factors, including injury.
- Metastatic disease to lower spine
- Leptomeningeal disease with advanced malignancy
- Lumbosacral plexopathy either from tumor or after radiation
- Vascular insufficiency

History

- Potential symptoms with involved tumors include:
  - Lumbosacral pain
  - Radiation of pain into buttocks and groin
  - Worse pain with prolonged sitting
  - Saddle numbness through perirectal and scrotal area
  - Constipation
  - Difficulty voiding
  - Sexual dysfunction
  - Gait may be affected.

Examination

- Potential findings with tumors in sacral region include:
  - Motor/sensory deficits in sacral nerve roots, including weakness about the ankles.
  - Gait abnormality

Testing

- Sacral mass on MRI with possible involvement of bone, neural foramina, and soft tissue

Treatment

- Aggressive multidisciplinary rehabilitation in the inpatient setting is very helpful.
- Requires close interaction with surgical services involved, especially plastic surgery.
  - The joint range-of-motion and weight-bearing restrictions should be clarified with plastic surgery service regularly.
  - Communication regarding such restrictions and updating functional goals to reflect such changes are of paramount importance.
- Pain management can be quite difficult and initially patients need intravenous patient-controlled analgesia.
  - Use of adjuvant agents is frequent.
  - Pain can vary with functional activities and a pretherapy analgesic regimen is frequently required.
  - Consultation with pain service is helpful for not only managing the inpatient pain but gradual titration of analgesic regimen in the outpatient setting.
- Median length of stay—18.5 days in nonrectal cancer patients

Prognosis

- Complications are frequent and are more common with a larger tumor size at the time of presentation.
- With myocutaneous flap, hospital stay increases several fold to ensure optimal clinical and functional outcome (from 8.5 days without flap to 36.5 days with flap).
- Bowel and bladder function:
  - More cephalad levels of resection are associated with significantly worse bowel and bladder control.

- Bowel incontinence lengthens hospital stay (39 days with versus 8 days without):
  - Wound-healing duration increases with bowel incontinence (93.5 days with versus 34 days without).
- Strong correlation between S3 nerve root integrity and continence:
  - Bilateral S3 intact—25% with bowel incontinence
  - Unilateral S3 intact—37.5% with bowel incontinence
  - Bilateral S3 resection—75% with bowel incontinence
  - Bowel and bladder functions are closely related.
- Ambulation is preserved in more than half of the patients with unilateral or bilateral S1 nerve root sacrifice.
- The majority of nonrectal cancer patients (more than 90%) can go home after rehabilitation.
- Tumor:
  - Tumor recurrence is not common and depends on the tumor.
    - With chordoma, mean time to metastasis: 50 months

Helpful Hints

- Management of sacrectomy patients is quite challenging, from both the surgical and rehabilitation perspectives.
- Frequent adjustments in functional restrictions means ongoing modifications in functional goals.
- Close coordination of care with surgical services and the nursing staff is needed.

Suggested Readings

Guo Y, Palmer JL, Shen L, et al. Bowel and bladder continence, wound healing, and functional outcomes in patients who underwent sacrectomy. *J Neurosurg Spine.* 2005;3:106–110.

Hsieh PC, Risheng X, Sciubba DM, et al. Long-term clinical outcomes following en bloc resections for sacral chordomas and chondrosarcomas. *Spine.* 2009;34:2233–2239.

Hulen CA, Temple HT, Fox WP, et al. Oncologic and functional outcome following sacrectomy for sacral chordoma. *J Bone Joint Surg Am,* 2006;88-A(7):1532–1539.

McPherson CM, Suki D, McCutcheon IE, et al. Metastatic disease from spinal chordoma: A 10-year experience. *J Neurosurg Spine.* 2006;5:277–280.

Schwab JH, Healey JH, Rose P, et al. The surgical management of sacral chordomas. *Spine.* 2009;34:2700–2704.

III: Cancer- or Treatment-Related Symptoms

Sexuality Issues

Mary K. Hughes MS RN CNS CT

Definition

Sexuality is a broad term, including social, emotional, and physical components. It includes body image, love of self and others, relating to others, and pleasure. It is genetically endowed, phenotypically embodied, hormonally nurtured, is not age related, and can be matured by experience. Sexuality includes affection, sexual orientation, sexual activity, eroticism, reproduction, intimacy, gender roles, and encompasses feelings of trust. It can contribute significantly to emotional well-being and overall satisfaction in life.

Etiology/Types

- Sexual dysfunction is failure of any aspect of the sexual-response cycle to function properly. Sexual concerns must be associated with distress to be considered a medical problem. A sexual problem includes:
  - Physiological dysfunction
  - Altered experiences
  - One's own perceptions and beliefs
  - Partner's perceptions and expectations
  - Altered circumstances
  - Past experiences
- Causes of sexual dysfunction in a person with cancer are often treatment related due to the changes in physiological, psychological, and social dimensions of sexuality and disruption in one or more phases of the sexual-response cycle. One of the greatest concerns of cancer survivors of childbearing age is the effect of treatment on fertility.

Epidemiology

- Up to 74% of patients with cancer experience some type of sexual dysfunction.
- Comorbidity of sexual dysfunctions is common.
- Almost half the men with low libido also have another sexual dysfunction.
- 20% of men with erectile dysfunction (ED) have low libido.

Pathogenesis

- Radiation and surgery can have longlasting effects on sexuality owing to chronic pain, scarring, and body-image issues.

- Besides chemotherapy, biologic agents, and hormones, there are numerous medications that can have sexual side effects that range from decreased desire to difficulty reaching orgasm.
- Low libido can be due to chemotherapy, menopause, hormone therapy, depression, pain, and anxiety.
- Arousal disorder (ED or vaginal dryness) can be due to irradiation, hormone therapy, surgery, menopause, depression, anxiety, and pain.
- Orgasmic difficulties can be due to surgery, irradiation, medications (SSRI), depression, pain, and anxiety.
- Dyspareunia can be due to vaginal dryness, inelasticity, shortening, or mucositis.

Risk Factors

- Men: after surgery for rectal or prostate cancer
- Irradiation to the pelvis, cranium, or total body
- Postmenopausal women, especially as a result of treatment
- Men and women on steroids, aromatase inhibitors, and androgen-deprivation therapy
- Poor body image
- Depression

Clinical Features

- Low libido
- Vaginal dryness, inelasticity, shortening
- Dyspareunia
- Erectile dysfunction
- Orgasm changes
- Ejaculatory problems
- Vaginismus

Diagnosis

History

- Onset may be sudden; preceding, during, or after treatment
- May improve after treatments are over
- May get worse after treatments are over
- Current medications
- Desire to conceive
- Type of cancer and treatments should be investigated
- Other treatment side effects should be investigated

- Ask, "What sexual changes have you noticed since…?"
- Probing questions:
  - How has your sexual desire changed?
  - Are you able to have erections? How firm?
    0 = no change, 1 = a bit larger, 2 = stuffable,
    3 = stickable, 4 = diamond cutter
  - Do you still have morning erections?
  - Do they last long enough to complete a sexual encounter?
  - Do you have vaginal dryness? What helps?
  - Are you able to have an orgasm?
    With or without partner? Have you ever had an orgasm?
  - How has this affected your relationship?

Examination
- Pelvic/genital exam
- Complete physical exam
  - Evaluate for neuropathy
  - Evaluate for vascular disease

Testing
- Hormone levels (testosterone, estradiol, thyroid)

Treatment
- Physical:
  - Vaginal lubricants (water soluble)
  - Vaginal moisturizers 2× week at night
  - Kegel exercises
  - Vaginal dilators
  - Erotic devices
  - L-arginine, an amino acid, anecdotally reported to improve arousal without stimulating estrogen production
  - Estrogen/testosterone replacement (topical or oral)
  - Thyroid replacement
  - Treat depression and anxiety
  - Treat pain and other symptoms
  - Pelvic floor therapist to help improve pelvic floor muscles
  - PDE5 inhibitors
  - Penile implants
  - Penile injections
  - Penile suppositories
  - Vacuum erection device
  - Fertility specialists
  - Reconstructive surgery
  - Breast implants
  - Contraceptive options
  - Physical therapy to improve endurance

- Behavioral:
  - Sensate-focus exercises with partner—begin touching each other in a sexual, but nonthreatening way. You tell them to focus on the receiver's pleasure and that there is to be no genital activity or sexual intercourse during this exercise. All of the senses are used.
  - Erotic lingerie
  - Erotic videos
  - Bibliotherapy
  - Ostomy appliance covers
  - Change sexual positions
  - Safer sex practices
  - Schedule sexual activity
  - Psychosexual therapy
  - Marital therapy
  - Stress reduction
- Fertility preservation:
  - Should be considered as early as possible during treatment.
  - Standard fertility preservation practice is:
    - Sperm cryopreservation for men
    - Embryo cryopreservation for women
    - Other methods considered investigational

Prognosis
- When treatments are over, some people notice a gradual improvement in sexual functioning. For others, improvement may take years, whereas others get worse over time. For many, their sexual functioning never returns to precancer functioning. The patient's partner and their relationship probably has a more profound effect on sexual health than any other factors.
- Many people have adopted a pattern of sexual behavior before their diagnosis and attempt to return to it after treatment. If they experience discomfort or failure to function as before, they will stop trying and feel they cannot enjoy sexual activity.
- Cancer survivors who are in a stressful relationship with an unsupportive partner can have more distress, leading to avoidant coping behaviors.

Helpful Hints
- Addressing possible sexual side effects of treatment helps prepare the patient for them.
- The patient feels validated when told that cancer treatment often has sexual side effects.
- Telling the patient that you are willing to help him/her improve sexual functioning gives them hope.

III: Cancer- or Treatment-Related Symptoms

- Using straightforward language and giving specific directions for using lubricants, moisturizers, and erotic devices helps patients understand what they need to do.
- Addressing sexuality in the first assessment lets the patient know that he or she is not the only one with sexual changes.
- Have a list of referrals in the community for marital therapy, psychiatric treatment, sexual counseling, and treatment.
- Get samples of vaginal lubricants and moisturizers to give to women so they can try them before they commit to buying.

- Get booklets from the American Cancer Society on cancer and sexuality to give to patients.
- Have available a list of reputable websites for patients to purchase erotic devices and lubricants.

Suggested Readings

Crenshaw TL, Goldberg JP. *Sexual Pharmacology: Drugs That Affect Sexual Functioning*. New York, NY: W. W. Norton; 1996.

Krebs LU. Sexual assessment in cancer care: Concepts, methods, and strategies for success. *Semin Oncol Nurs*. 2008;24(2):80–90.

Mulhall JP, Incrocci L, Goldstein I, et al, eds. *Cancer and Sexual Health*. New York, NY: Humana Press; 2011.

Sleep Disorders

Saadia A. Faiz MD ▪ Lara Bashoura MD ▪ Diwakar Balachandran MD

Description

Sleep-related complaints, such as insomnia, fatigue, and daytime sleepiness, are common complaints in cancer patients. Sleep disturbances may be due to a primary underlying sleep disorder, current therapy, underlying anxiety and/or mood disorder, or sequelae of other medical conditions, or the cancer itself. Although some studies have used actigraphy and polysomnography (PSG), research in this area has been primarily descriptive and survey based. Poor sleep may be an important predictor of decreased quality of life, and it may impact energy level, mood, and participation in rehabilitation.

Etiology/Types

- Insomnia: difficulty initiating and/or maintaining sleep, early-morning awakenings, and resultant deficit in daytime function. There are several types of insomnia:
  - Acute insomnia (after inciting event)
  - Psychophysiological insomnia:
    - Psychophysiological insomnia is one of the most common types of insomnia, in which symptoms persist long after the precipitating event.
  - Inadequate sleep hygiene:
    - Inadequate sleep hygiene refers to sleeping in an environment or participating in rituals not conducive to sleep.
- Sleep-related breathing disorders: abnormal respiratory pattern (apneas, hypopneas, or respiratory effort-related arousals) or hypoventilation during sleep. Obstructive sleep has an increased incidence in men and in postmenopausal women, obesity, middle age, family history, and physical characteristics including large neck, facial and skull abnormalities, enlarged tonsils.
  - Sleep-related hypoventilation is usually presumed when persistent oxygen desaturation is noted during sleep, and potential causes could include obesity hypoventilation syndrome, pulmonary parenchymal or vascular pathology, lower airway obstruction and neuromuscular and chest wall disorders.
- Movement disorders: usually refers to restless legs syndrome (RLS) or periodic limb movements of sleep (PLMS). Workup aside from clinical history includes evaluation of laboratory data to exclude electrolyte abnormalities, anemia, iron deficiency, poor glycemic control, and thyroid dysfunction. May also be associated with significant caffeine intake.

Epidemiology

- The true prevalence of sleep complaints may vary on the basis of the cancer, current therapy, and other comorbidities.
- In one study of a broad base of cancer types, the most prevalent problems were:
  - Excessive fatigue (44%)
  - Leg restlessness (41%)
  - Insomnia (31%)
  - Excessive sleepiness (28%)
- Future research may elucidate the true prevalence, but there is likely significant variation based on underlying malignancy and treatment.

Risk Factors

- Insomnia: Higher rates of insomnia have been reported in patients with cancer compared to the general population. The development of insomnia in the general population and in cancer groups has been associated with:
  - Female gender
  - Advanced age
  - Anxiety
  - Depression
  - Medical comorbidities
- Sleep-disordered breathing:
  - Obstructive sleep apnea has been described with increased incidence in head and neck cancer patients, so these patients in particular should be screened.
  - Chronic opioid usage may also be associated with central sleep apnea or more complex sleep-related breathing disturbance.
- Movement disorder:
  - Anemia is common in cancer patients, either related to the underlying malignancy or to the therapy; it may precipitate symptoms of RLS.

III: Cancer- or Treatment-Related Symptoms

125

Diagnosis

Differential diagnosis

- Psychological and psychiatric:
  - High prevalence of psychological distress, sleep disruption, and related factors among cancer patients.
  - Sleep symptoms may hallmark an underlying mood disorder.
  - Early-morning awakenings, excessive daytime fatigue, insomnia, and nocturnal awakenings may be manifestations of depression or anxiety disorders.
- Pain:
  - Often contributes to the development and persistence of sleep disruption.
  - Sleep deprivation may also lower pain threshold.
- Cancer-related fatigue: Fatigue may occur before diagnosis, during treatment, and for years after cancer-related therapy is completed. Contributing factors include:
  - Anemia (most common)
  - Physical deconditioning
  - Medications
  - Cachexia
  - Poor nutrition
  - Endocrinopathies
- Medication side effects:
  - Pain and antiepileptic medications may cause daytime hypersomnia.
  - Titration of selective serotonin receptor antagonists may also exacerbate movement disorders.
- Neuropathy:
  - May create symptoms similar to movement disorders.
- Comorbidities: Other medical conditions can disrupt sleep.
  - Gastroesophageal reflux
  - Cardiomyopathy
  - Menopause
  - Rheumatologic disorders such as fibromyalgia may also contribute to sleep disruption if not optimized.

Testing

- Sleep diaries: The patient completes a 2-week diary that includes information regarding caffeine intake, exercise, medication, alcohol intake, type of day (work, school, vacation, weekend), naps, and sleep schedule (sleep time, wake time). Review of the diary provides a visual tool of the patient's sleep cycle and clues as to the etiology of the sleep disturbance.
- Surveys:
  - The Pittsburgh Sleep Quality Index (PSQI) is the most widely used sleep-specific questionnaire; it measures subjective sleep quality during the previous month.
  - The Epworth Sleepiness Scale assesses daytime sleepiness; a positive score (10 or higher) often prompts evaluation for underlying sleep disorder with PSG.
- PSG: It is the gold standard for diagnosis of sleep-disordered breathing. A comprehensive PSG includes computerized polygraph to monitor electroencephalogram, electrooculogram, electrocardiogram, chin and anterior tibialis electromyogram, abdominal and chest wall excursion using impedance plethysmography, airflow by nasal pressure and nasal and oral thermistors, and oxygen saturation (SaO_2) by pulse oximetry. A positive pressure titration study involves PSG with titration of positive pressure therapy to eliminate snoring and sleep disordered breathing.
- Actigraphy: Actigraphy is a noninvasive method of monitoring human rest and activity cycles. It measures gross motor activity, and can be useful in determining sleep patterns and circadian rhythms.

Treatment

- Insomnia: Treatment for insomnia consists of both pharmacologic treatment and psychological and behavioral therapies.
  - Cognitive-behavioral therapy (CBT) is indicated for all patients with insomnia. CBT may be administered alone or in combination with hypnotic medications. Education in proper sleep hygiene including regularization of sleep timings, maintaining an optimal sleeping environment, avoiding use of bed for activities other than sleep, and restricting caffeine are standard practices to improve sleep quality.
- Sleep-disordered breathing:
  - Patients with sleep apnea are treated with positive pressure therapy.
  - Patients with sleep-related hypoventilation may require supplemental oxygen with sleep.
  - Concomitant disorders such as chronic obstructive pulmonary disease, asthma, interstitial lung disease, and cardiac disorders should also be optimized.

■ Movement disorder:
  – Treatment of underlying metabolic disorders is the first-line therapy, followed by elimination of caffeine.
  – Pharmacologic treatment includes dopamine agonists.

Helpful Hints

■ Sleep disorders are common but often unrecognized in cancer patients.

■ Insomnia is the most common sleep disorder in cancer patients.

■ Sleep disorders may arise as a result of cancer or cancer-related therapies.

■ Primary sleep disorders such as insomnia, sleep-disordered breathing, and limb movements should be evaluated in cancer patients with sleep complaints. Investigations may include screening tools including surveys and laboratory studies, and if necessary referral to a sleep specialist and polysomnography should be considered.

■ Treatment of sleep disorders may involve cognitive and behavior therapy and sleep hygiene for insomnia, positive airway pressure for sleep apnea, oxygen for sleep-related hypoventilation, or pharmacologic therapy for limb movement disorders.

Suggested Readings

Davidson JR, MacLean AW, Brundage MD, Schulze K. Sleep disturbance in cancer patients. *Soc Sci Med.* 2002;54:1309–1321.

Parish JM. Sleep-related problems in common medical conditions. *Chest.* 2009;135:563–572.

Sateia M, Lang BJ. Sleep and cancer: Recent developments. *Curr Oncol Rep.* 2008;10:309–318.

Stepanski EJ, Burgess HJ. Sleep and cancer. *Sleep Med Clin.* 2007;2:67–75.

Spasticity

Jack B. Fu MD

Description
Velocity-dependent resistance to range-of-motion (ROM) movement of a joint.

Etiology/Types
- Spasticity is caused by an upper motor neuron injury.
- Severity is typically graded using the Modified Ashworth Scale:
  - 0: No spasticity
  - 1: Slight increase in resistance to ROM, not sustained
  - 2: Increased tone throughout ROM, but affected part(s) easily moved
  - 3: Passive movement difficult
  - 4: Affected part(s) rigid

Epidemiology
- Most commonly seen in the cancer population in patients with primary brain tumors, particularly astrocytomas and meningiomas.
- May be the consequence of tumor itself and/or radiation effects.
- Many of the spasticity patients who present to a cancer rehabilitation clinic are cancer patients who have had strokes.
- The frequency of spasticity in cancer patients is not well studied but appears to be less than in patients with other central nervous system (CNS) injury etiologies.

Pathogenesis
- After upper motor neuron damage, there is decreased cortical inhibition of the stretch reflex.
- Results in increased velocity-dependent resistance to movement.

Risk Factors
- CNS tumor
- The longer the patient's history of CNS tumor, the more likely he or she is to have spasticity. This can be due to the increased likelihood of CNS damage from radiation and surgeries.
- History of radiation necrosis

Clinical Features
- Velocity-dependent increase in resistance to passive range of motion

- Clonus
- Hyperreflexia

Diagnosis

Differential diagnosis
- Soft tissue contracture
- Parkinsonism

History
- History of upper motor neuron damage, followed by a progressive increase in resistance to passive movement
- Patient with a known history of CNS tumor
- Postresection patients likely have a "shock" period for several weeks before the onset of spasticity.
- Patients may develop spasticity months after radiation treatment owing to radiation late effects.
- Gradual increase in tone follows.

Examination
- Can be characterized by a "catch" resistance noted by the examiner.
- The resistance experienced by examiner will be velocity dependent.
- Modified Ashworth scale should be used to quantify the spasticity.

Pitfalls
- Any cancer patient who develops new spasticity should be evaluated to establish a source for the symptom.

Treatment

Medical
- A number of oral antispasmodic agents can be given, including baclofen, diazepam, dantrolene, and tizanidine. The limiting factor is oversedation.

Injections
- Botulinum toxin injections can achieve effects for 2 to 6 months.
- Phenol and alcohol neurolysis injections can result in effects lasting 6 to 12 months.

Implantable pumps

- Intrathecal baclofen pumps can be used.
- Many cancer patients with chronic pain have implanted intrathecal pain pumps. Baclofen can be used in a mixture with their analgesic medications.
  - Benefits include the ability to titrate baclofen doses and minimize sedation effects.
  - Negative factors include cost, pump-related side effects, and the need for implantation.

Therapy/exercises

- Stretching and ROM exercises can decrease spasticity and prevent soft tissue contracture formation.
- Serial casting and stretch splints can also reduce tone and improve ROM in combination with other treatments.
- Positioning of the affected extremity through the use of splints may help prevent contracture formation.
- Surgical procedures, although rarely used, include tendon lengthening.

Consults

- Physical medicine and rehabilitation
- Neurology
- Pain management or neurosurgery for intrathecal baclofen pump implantation

Complications of treatment

- Antispasticity medications can cause potential sedation, hypotension, dependence, and withdrawal issues.

- Antibody resistance to injectable medications can develop.
- Intrathecal baclofen pump malfunction can occur with the risk of worsening tone and withdrawal.
- Muscle atrophy and excessive weakness can develop from treatment.

Prognosis

- Untreated spasticity can lead to soft tissue contracture and functional decline.

Helpful Hints

- Many cancer patients suffer from pancytopenia from cancer treatment. Check blood cell counts and coagulation studies before pursuing injections or device implantation.
- Botulinum toxin injection can be used for comfort care in patients with a limited prognosis for pain reduction and to assist caregivers with positioning.
- Similar to the nononcologic population, spasticity can worsen with infection.

Suggested Readings

Dones I, Nazzi V, Broggi G. The guidelines for the diagnosis and treatment of spasticity. *J Neurosurg Sci.* 2006;50(4):101–105.

Rekand T. Clinical assessment and management of spasticity: A review. *Acta Neurol Scand Suppl.* 2010;(190):62–66.

Sheean G. The pathophysiology of spasticity. *Eur J Neurol.* 2002;9(S1):3–9.

Steroid Myopathy

Ying Guo MD MS

Description

Myopathy, a well-recognized side effect of systemic glucocorticoid (corticosteroid) therapy, can occur with any of the glucocorticoid preparations.

Etiology

- Muscle weakness due to muscle wasting and atrophy caused by corticosteroid use
- Several cancer patient populations are frequently exposed to glucocorticoid treatment:
  – Lymphoma
  – Bone marrow transplant patients
  – Bone marrow transplant with graft-versus-host disease
  – Patients with primary or secondary brain or spinal cord tumor
  – Palliative care patients

Epidemiology

- Daily doses in excess of 40 to 60 mg/day (prednisone equivalent) can induce clinically significant weakness within 2 weeks and almost always result in some degree of muscle weakness when continued for 1 month or more.

Pathogenesis

- Intracellular glucocorticoid receptors are important in the etiology of steroid myopathy.
- Myocyte apoptosis
- May decrease muscle cell differentiation

Risk Factors

- Older age
- Malnutrition
- Cancer
- Higher dose of glucocorticoid more likely to develop steroid myopathy
- Fluorinated form of corticosteroid is more likely to cause myopathy.

Clinical Features

- Lower extremity proximal weakness usually occurs before upper extremity weakness and is more severe.
- Can cause difficulty in getting up from a chair/toilet, climbing stairs, or performing overhead tasks.
- Decreased balance, increased risk for falls
- Some patients develop respiratory muscle weakness, which may lead to respiratory dysfunction.

Diagnosis

Differential diagnosis

- Inflammatory myopathy: increase in serum muscle enzyme and a lack of other features related to corticosteroid use. Electromyogram (EMG) shows signs of muscle membrane instability such as fibrillation and positive sharp waves. Muscle biopsy can also provide further evidence for differential diagnosis.
- Critical illness myopathy: severe diffuse proximal and distal weakness. EMG shows normal- to low-amplitude motor nerve conduction study and normal- or near-normal sensory nerve conduction study. Needle electromyography may not always reveal fibrillation potential activity; depending on the degree of weakness, the recruitment of motor unit potentials (MUPs) may be difficult. Motor unit potentials are short in duration, low in amplitude.

History

- Gradual onset, usually after use of corticosteroid
- Progressive disability and worsening performance status are associated with muscle weakness.

Examination

- Muscle strength is usually decreased in hip flexor and hip extensor muscle groups, sometimes present in the shoulder abductors and flexors. Distal muscle strength is less affected.
- Myalgias and muscle tenderness are not observed.

Treatment

- Discontinue steroid if possible.
- Decrease steroid dose to lowest possible.
- Change to nonfluorinated form of steroid if possible.
- Accommodate the hip weakness by providing higher transfer surfaces with a cushion, raised toilet, and lift chair.

Prognosis

- Short-term inpatient rehabilitation combined with reduction of steroid dose is effective in improving functional status.

Helpful Hints

- Patient's strength can improve within 1 week after steroid is discontinued.
- In situations in which steroid must be continued, use compensatory strategies such as higher transfer surfaces and other assistive devices.

Suggested Readings

Bowyer SL, LaMothe MP, Hollister JR. Steroid myopathy: Incidence and detection in a population with asthma. *J Allergy Clin Immunol.* 1985;76(2 Pt 1):234.

Dropcho EJ, Soong SJ. Steroid-induced weakness in patients with primary brain tumors. *Neurology.* 1991;41(8): 1235.

Konagaya M, Bernard PA, Max SR. Blockade of glucocorticoid receptor binding and inhibition of dexamethasone-induced muscle atrophy in the rat by RU38486, a potent glucocorticoid antagonist. *Endocrinology.* 1986;119(1):375.

Mercadante SL, Berchovich M, Casuccio A, et al. A prospective randomized study of corticosteroids as adjuvant drugs to opioids in advanced cancer patients. *Am J Hosp Palliat Care.* 2007;24(1):13.

Thromboembolic Disease and Prophylaxis

Amy Ng MD MPH

Description

Venous thromboembolism (VTE) most commonly forms in the veins of the lower extremities or thighs (deep venous thrombosis or DVT). It can present as pulmonary embolism (PE) obstructing the pulmonary artery or in an arterial branch leading to the lungs. VTE is the second leading cause of death in cancer patients. It is a significant predictor of mortality in hospitalized patients with cancer.

Etiology

- Formation of a blood clot in the venous blood vessels in the absence of bleeding in the veins of the legs or extremities (DVT) or lungs (PE).

Epidemiology

- 2% to 25% of patients with idiopathic VTE are found to have cancer within 24 months of the diagnosis of VTE.
- Certain sites of cancer have a higher risk of VTE:
  - Pancreas
  - Stomach
  - Brain
  - Ovary
  - Lung
  - Metastatic disease
- Hematological malignancies, including lymphoma, leukemia, and myeloma, have relatively high rates of VTE.
- The relative risk of developing VTE is approximately seven times higher in patients with active cancer, with a higher incidence rate in the first 30 to 60 days after cancer diagnosis.
- In a retrospective cohort study among over one million cancer patients from 1995 to 2003, the overall VTE rate was 4.1%; 3.4% were diagnosed with DVT and 1.1% with PE.

Pathogenesis

- Virchow's triad:
  - Hypercoagulable state
  - Venous injury
  - Venous stasis
- Cancer patients are in a hypercoagulable state and are more prone to venous stasis as result of immobility due to illness.

- Venous thrombi consist of deposits of fibrin, red cells, platelets, and leukocytes.
  - Thrombi usually begin to form at low-flow sites.
  - Platelets interact with subendothelial constituents and initiate thrombus formation with activation of coagulation factors.
  - Clearance of activated coagulation factors is prevented by venous stasis and facilitates interactions of thrombus with the vessel wall.
  - The relative balance between activated coagulation and the thrombolytic system determines further propagation and dissolution of thrombus.

Risk Factors for Venous Thromboembolism

- Immobility during acute illness
- Fractures
- Prior history of thromboembolism
- Heart failure
- Obesity
- Age over 70 years
- Pregnancy or estrogen therapy

Clinical Features

- May be asymptomatic and without any clinical signs
- May have redness, pain, or swelling in the limbs
- DVT may progress and travel to the lungs, leading to PE.

Diagnosis

Differential diagnosis

- DVT:
  - Superficial phlebitis
  - Cellulitis
  - Fracture
  - Arterial occlusion
  - Edema
- PE:
  - Pneumonia
  - Myocardial infarction
  - Pneumothorax
  - Gastroesophageal reflux disease (GERD)

History
- Immobility
- Acute illness
- Hypercoagulable state
- Family history of thrombosis, sudden death

Examination
- Often unremarkable
- May have swelling, pain, redness in legs

Testing
- Doppler ultrasound of suspected limb
- Spiral CT of lungs
- Ventilation-perfusion scan
- D-dimer elevation

Pitfalls
- Patients may be asymptomatic.
- Doppler ultrasound may not visualize all veins of the extremity.
  - Sensitivity for proximal DVT is high (94.2%) but is low (63.5%) for nonoccluding or isolated calf thrombi.
  - If clinical concern remains despite negative results, repeat or serial ultrasound studies in 7 to 14 days.
- Ventilation-perfusion scan may be inconclusive.

Red Flags
- Tachycardia
- Shortness of breath, hypoxia
- Chest pain
- Bleeding
- Pain in legs

Treatment

Medical
- Prophylaxis:
  - Current consensus guidelines of the American College of Chest Physicians and the American Society of Clinical Oncology recommend thromboprophylaxis with low-molecular-weight heparin (LMWH; grade 1A), low-dose unfractionated heparin (LDUH; grade 1A), or fondaparinux (grade 1A) for cancer patients who are bedridden with an acute medical illness.
  - Routine use of thromboprophylaxis for primary prevention of VTE is not recommended for cancer patients receiving chemotherapy or hormonal therapy (grade 1C).
- Treatment of established VTE:
  - Cancer-associated thrombosis treatment includes LMWH for 3 to 6 months (grade 1A) followed by Vitamin K antagonists such as Coumadin or LMWH for an indefinite duration for those with active malignancy or ongoing treatment for cancer (grade 1C).
  - LMWH reduces the risk of VTE recurrence up to 50%, as shown in randomized controlled trials.
  - Inferior vena cava (IVC) filter may further help to reduce the risk of PE but it does not decrease the risk of DVT formation.

Exercises
- Early mobilization
- Passive range of motion

Consults
- Vascular surgery or interventional radiology for IVC filter placement.

Complications of treatment
- Increased bleeding risk, especially in renal impairment; up to three to six times greater risk
- Heparin-induced thrombocytopenia
- Difficult management of Coumadin depending on comorbid conditions, interactions with chemotherapy, antibiotics, or poor nutrition
- Skin infection or sensitivity at site of injection
- Migration of IVC filter

Prognosis
- Poor, if VTE is left untreated
- Approximately one third of patients treated for cancer-associated VTE die within 3 months after VTE diagnosis.
- Patients diagnosed with cancer within 1 year of VTE also have a higher prevalence of metastatic disease and reduced survival, compared with cancer patients without VTE.

Helpful Hints
- Physical therapy, including mobilization and range of motion, can begin after anticoagulation is initiated.
- Routine noninvasive screening for DVT with Doppler ultrasound should be considered for patients not already on thromboembolic prophylaxis.

Suggested Readings
Babu B, Carman TL. Cancer and clots: All cases of venous thromboembolism are not treated the same. *Cleve Clin J Med.* 2009;76(2):129–135.

Braddom RL. *Physical Medicine and Rehabilitation.* 4th ed. Philadelphia, PA: Elsevier Saunders; 2011;1358–1365.

Geerts WH, Bergqvist D, Pineo GF, et al. American society of clinical oncology guideline: Recommendations for venous thromboembolism prophylaxis and treatment in patients with cancer. *J Clin Oncol.* 2007;25(24):5490–5505.

Khorana AA, Francis CW, Culakova E, et al. Frequency, risk factors, and trends for venous thromboembolism among hospitalized cancer patients. *Cancer.* 2007;110(10):2339–2346.

Wun T, White RH. Epidemiology of cancer-related venous thromboembolism. *Best Pract Res Clin Haematol.* 2009;22:9–23.

III: Cancer- or Treatment-Related Symptoms

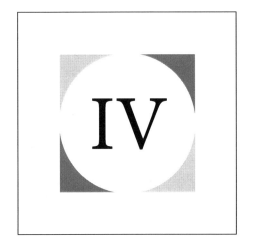

Special Concerns

Advanced Care Planning and Advance Directives

Donna S. Zhukovsky MD FACP FAAHPM

Description

Ms. PT is a 53-year-old elementary school teacher with advanced metastatic breast cancer. She is hospitalized on your acute rehabilitation unit to maximize function after surgery done to relieve spinal cord compression. One night, Ms. PT develops respiratory insufficiency and delirium and is transferred to the intensive care unit for stabilization. She last saw her husband 5 years ago; her three adult children have not been involved in her care. She has been living with her oldest brother and is close to most of her seven siblings, many of whom have been present throughout her stay on the rehabilitation unit. How aggressive should you be with her care and to whom should you turn for assistance with medical decision making?

Advance Care Planning

- Advance care planning is a process by which individuals can plan for future health care in the event of decisional incapacity.
- Advance care planning:
  - Can begin anywhere along the health care continuum, including with people who do not have known health conditions
  - Is closely related to the concepts of patient autonomy and self-determination
  - Is predicated on expert communication among the individual and the individual's surrogate decision maker and clinicians
- Meaningful advance care planning requires:
  - Understanding, reflecting, and discussing the individual's health state and care options in the context of his or her values and goals
  - Formulating and documenting a plan
  - Communicating the plan to involved loved ones and the medical team
  - Reviewing the plan periodically to ensure that it remains consistent with values and goals, especially with changes in health condition
  - Enacting the plan under the appropriate circumstances

- Most patients prefer advance care planning:
  - To be initiated by their physician
  - To occur in the outpatient setting
  - To take place during periods of relative stability
- Advance care planning:
  - Does *not* typically result in increased distress for patients or surrogate decision makers
  - *Is* associated with fewer bereavement complications for surrogate decision makers

Advance Directives

Advance directives are documents that convey information about advance care plans.

- Types of advance directives include:
  - Instructional documents, more commonly known as directives or living wills, that indicate a person's preferences for health care received in certain health states
  - Documents that designate a surrogate decision maker during periods of incapacity for medical decision making. These documents are variously known as a Medical Power of Attorney, Durable Power of Attorney for Health Care or Health Care Proxy.
  - Physician order forms that convert patient preferences into medical orders, such as out of hospital do not resuscitate order forms (OOH DNR) or more broadly based forms such as physician orders for life-sustaining therapy (POLST) and medical orders for life-sustaining therapy (MOLST) forms. Some of these forms require patient signatures as well as a physician signature. Their availability varies from state to state.
- Advance directives may be *statutory* or *advisory*. Statutory documents are based on legal requirements codified in state law. Not all states have statutory forms for instructional documents and those that designate a surrogate decision maker. However, states will often honor statutory documents from other states. Advisory documents not codified in state law also carry legal weight if they provide clear evidence of the patient's wishes.

- If a person does not designate a surrogate decision maker and need arises, the selection is based on a legal hierarchy determined by each state. For married individuals, the responsible party is usually the spouse, irrespective of separation or estrangement.

Choice of a Surrogate Decision Maker

- When discussing the choice of a surrogate decision maker with the patient:
  - Emphasize selection of an agent who is familiar with the person's values and goals for health care, and how they influence care preferences.
  - Confirm willingness of the proposed surrogate decision maker to accept the responsibility of the role.
  - Involve the surrogate decision maker in advance care planning discussions.
  - Ascertain the surrogate's ability to make decisions based on the patient's wishes and not his or her own personal wishes.
  - Clarify the degree of flexibility the patient grants the surrogate decision maker in the decision-making process. Does the patient want that person to follow the patient's stated preferences precisely or does the patient allow the decision maker the discretion to deviate from previously articulated preferences, based on what he or she thinks would be best at the time?

Helpful Hints

- Incorporate advance care planning systematically into the care of your patients.

- Introduce the topic in the outpatient setting at a time of relative stability, whenever possible.
- Emphasize that you would like to understand his or her concerns and what is important to him or her, in the event that complications arise. Also encourage the individual to bring his or her surrogate decision maker with him or her to the appointment, so that the surrogate may also better understand the patient's values and goals for future health care.
- Ensure transparency of advance care plan and availability of advance directives in all care settings.
- Revisit the care plan periodically, especially with changes in the individual's health status, to ascertain consistency with current values and goals for health care.

Suggested Readings

Fins JJ, Maltby BS, Friedmann E, et al. Contracts, covenants and advance care planning: An empirical study of the moral obligations of patient and proxy. *J Pain Symptom Manage.* 2005;29(1):55–68.

Sudore RL, Fried TR. Redefining the "planning" in advance care planning: Preparing for end-of-life decision making. *Ann Intern Med.* 2010;153(4):256–261.

Wendler D, Rid A. Systematic review: The effect on surrogates on making treatment decisions for others. *Ann Intern Med.* 2011;154(5):336–346.

Zhukovsky DS, Bruera E. A transcultural perspective of advanced directives in palliative care. In: *Palliative Medicine.* London, UK: Edward Arnold Ltd.; 2006: 1035–1043.

IV: Special Concerns

Alcohol Use in the Cancer Patient

Kathie Rickman DrPH RN CNS

Description

- Alcohol is the most commonly abused substance in America:
  - 75,000 deaths per year are related to alcohol use.
  - 600,000 injuries and 800,000 assaults per year are alcohol related.
  - 24% of suicides in the United States are related to alcohol use.
  - Researchers have linked alcohol consumption to more than 60 diseases/conditions.
  - Alcohol is considered a poison by the body; all efforts go toward excreting it.
- In May 2000, alcohol was added to the list of human carcinogens in the National Toxicology Program Report to the U.S. Department of Health and Human Services.
- Research has established the relationship between consumption of alcohol and certain cancers:
  - Strong associations with mouth, esophageal, laryngeal, pharyngeal, breast, and liver cancers.
  - Drinkers who smoke are at even higher risk for these cancers.
  - Risks increase with amount of alcohol consumed; highest among heavy drinkers.
  - Even a few drinks a week may increase a person's risk.
  - Women who are undergoing hormone replacement therapy and who drink just *one drink* per day *double* their chances of developing breast cancer.
- Drinking alcohol during cancer treatment is not recommended because:
  - Alcohol is metabolized by the liver as are many chemotherapies and medications.
  - Alcohol can interfere with the liver's ability to effectively metabolize toxins such as chemotherapeutic agents.
  - Alcohol interacts with many prescribed and over-the-counter medications to cause harmful effects/outcomes.
  - Alcohol has a dehydrating effect and may contribute to electrolyte losses.
  - Alcohol may irritate mouth sores caused by chemotherapy.

- Alcohol and seniors:
  - Alcohol and substance abuse are statistically at *epidemic* proportions among the elderly and remain mostly unreported.
  - Seniors purchase the majority of over-the-counter and prescription medications; they are at risk for serious, sometimes *fatal drug interactions* when combining alcohol with medications. Patients are strongly advised to refrain from drinking and combining *any medication,* including chemotherapeutic agents, with alcohol.

Assessment

- It is important to assess for alcohol use or abuse as this is a potential risk to treatment outcomes:
  - CAGE Questionnaire
  - Quantity–frequency: x days a week × number of drinks per day × 4 weeks = TOTAL/month. If more than 60 drinks a month for males and more than 30 drinks a month for females, there is an increased risk for problem drinking. May need a detoxification program before treatment starts (National Institute on Alcohol Abuse and Alcoholism Standards).

History

- Previous treatment: detoxification, Alcoholics Anonymous attendance, residential rehabilitation
- Family history: first- and second-degree relatives with alcoholism
- Legal issues related to use: driving while intoxicated (DWI), public intoxication, probation
- Medical sequelae: cirrhosis, hypertension, falls with or without injuries
- Social issues: relationship discord, job loss, avoidance of friends/family
- History of liver diseases related to alcohol:
  - Fatty liver
  - Alcoholic hepatitis
  - Cirrhosis

Cancer-Related Issues

- Caution with chemotherapy in the presence of liver disease:

 – Patients undergoing cytotoxic chemotherapy require careful assessment of liver function both prior to and during therapy. Potential interactions between the liver and chemotherapy fall into three categories:
   • Direct chemotherapy-induced hepatotoxicity
   • Worsening of preexisting liver disease, especially viral hepatitis
   • Altered metabolism and excretion of chemotherapy drugs cleared by the liver can result in increased systemic toxicity (particularly myelosuppression) or worsening of chemotherapy-induced hepatotoxicity.
■ Best practices during cancer treatment:
 – Abstinence from alcohol of all types
 – Treatment of underlying withdrawal and/or anxiety with benzodiazepines
 – Relapse prevention; monitor sleep, mood symptoms, and triggers to relapse
 – Treat symptoms of depression, anxiety, insomnia

Suggested Readings

American Cancer Society. http://www.cancer.gov

American Institute for Cancer Research. May, 2008. Newsletter. http://www.aicr.org

Bagnardi V, Blangiardo M, La Vecchia C, Corrao G. Alcohol consumption and the risk of cancer: A meta-analysis. *Alcohol Res Health*. 2001;25(4):263–270.

Buddy T. Ignoring the problem of senior substance abuse: Doctors reluctant to make diagnosis. *Alcoholism Newsletter*, July, 2006: About.com

Centers for Disease Control and Prevention. Alcohol and suicide among racial/ethnic populations. *MMWR Morb Mortal Wkly Rep*. 2009;58(23):637–641.

Chen WY, Colditz GA, Rosner B, et al. Use of postmenopausal hormones, alcohol, and risk for invasive breast cancer. *Ann Int Med*. 2002;137:798–804.

National Institute on Alcohol Abuse and Alcoholism. http://www.niaaa.nih.gov

Savarese, D. Chemotherapy Hepatotoxicity and Dose Modification in Patients with Liver Disease. http://www.uptodate.com. Topic last updated: March 29, 2012.

IV: Special Concerns

Difficult Conversations

Walter Baile MD

Description

Difficult conversations include giving bad news, dealing with patient and family emotions, and answering questions such as "will I get better?"

Breaking Bad News—Key Points

Definition

- Any information that seriously threatens to change the outlook of one's future
- Types of bad news:
  - Discussing a serious disorder or diagnosis
  - Warning about the unlikelihood that treatment will help
  - Ending a treatment without resolution of the disease

Challenges in giving bad news

- Having a strategy
- Avoiding allowing one's own emotions to come into play
- Knowing how to address the patient's reaction to bad news

S-P-I-K-E-S: A 6-step strategy for giving bad news

- S = Get the setting right:
  - Don't have the conversation in the hallway.
  - Take precautions not to be interrupted (e.g., phone silenced).
  - Have the right people in the room (whoever the patient wants to be there).
- P = Prepare:
  - Know what the status of the patient is (review medical and other findings).
  - Have a plan for the patient.
  - If the news is really bad, think about how the patient might react and how you will deal with that.
- I = Invitation:
  - Make sure the patient is ready (don't give bad news when the patient does not want it, is in pain, sedated, or the right people are not in the room; "is it ok if we discuss…").
- K = Knowledge:
  - Before giving information, check and see how much the patient already knows and expects (if he or she seems to know what's coming, the task is easier than when it is a complete surprise).
  - Chunk information: give it in blocks and check whether the patient has understood.
  - Avoid using jargon: even phrases such as "nerve stimulation" might be beyond the patient's comprehension.
- E = Address emotion:
  - Be ready for emotions as they are a common reaction to bad news, and they are a normal human way of expressing disappointment, frustration, or anxiety.
  - Try to avoid reacting to patient emotions right away or with a "reassurance" or promise that things will get better.
  - Respond to emotions with an empathic response that simply acknowledges emotions. This will help patients recover and allows them to begin to ask questions about "what's next?" Examples of empathic statements include:
    - "I can see this really knocked you for a loop."
    - "I can see you weren't expecting this."
    - "Most people in your shoes would be upset also."
  - Avoid saying:
    - "I can feel your pain" (you can't).
    - "This will get better" (you don't know).
    - "I understand how you feel" (you can't).
  - Don't take it personally if patients get angry at you or the system or blame somebody. He or she is most likely feeling helpless, frightened, or demoralized.
- S = Strategy and summary:
  - Leave the patient and family with a plan (be aware that most of what you say may not be remembered so…).
  - Check to see what they understood ("Can you tell me what you understand?").
  - Send a summary letter.
    - **Pearl:** This paradigm can be used to discuss prognosis, advanced directives, and end-of-life conversations.

Other Types of Difficult Conversations

When the patient is in denial

- Denial is often a temporary form of disbelief and a reaction to shocking information. "I can't believe this is happening to me"; "Are you sure there is no mistake?" Here, a "wish statement" may be indicated. "I wish it weren't true but unfortunately it is."

- Distortion may occur when the patient did not get the facts right or desires to cast the information in a better light. "Do you mean there is still a chance that it will get better?" This can also be answered with a wish statement such as "I wish it were possible."
- Deferral: "I just don't want to think about it now" is a commonly uttered phrase in response to feeling overwhelmed by a situation. In this case, the phrase "I can see you need more time" would be appropriate.
- Dismissal is a form of denial in which the statement of another person is devalued as not having credibility. It is often accompanied by anger toward another person. "I know that this can't be true. I want a second opinion." Again, the emotions behind the bad news are a request for more time to let the news sink in. Sometimes a second opinion will be a big help.

Difficult questions

Difficult questions are common in oncology. The key is to understand that behind the question there is often a concern.

- The patient who asks "how long do I have to live?" may be asking "am I going to make it to my daughter's graduation?"

- The patient who asks "will I suffer?" may have had the experience of seeing a loved one die without adequate pain control.
- The patient who asks "is there hope for me?" may want to know whether he or she should buy the condo in Florida he or she was saving for.

Helpful Hints

- With difficult questions it is always helpful to *explore* the reason for the question. "I'd be happy to answer your question but first it would help me to know how the information is going to help you."
- When patients ask "how long will it take for me to get better?" it is always useful to give ranges and not specific time periods as patients may vary greatly. "Most patients get better in 6 months but for others it takes a year."
- This is also true for patients who ask "how long do I have to live?" So first "explore," then "reveal."

Suggested Readings

Back A, Arnold R, Tulsky J. *Mastering Communications With Seriously Ill Patients*. New York, NY: Cambridge University Press; 2009.

Baile WF, Buckman R, Lenzi R, et al. SPIKES—A six-step protocol for delivering bad news: Application to the patient with cancer. *Oncologist*. 2000;5:302–311.

Lubinsky MS. Bearing bad news: Dealing with the mimics of denial. *Genet Counsel*. 1994;3:5–12.

Disability and the Return to Work in Cancer Patients

Benedict Konzen MD

Description

Employment is a rite of passage, usually representing a transition into adulthood. An adult is responsible for directing his or her financial security, establishing oneself in a career, and developing a family unit—and the inherent care responsibilities thereto. In the cancer patient, there are often unforeseen and unplanned disruptions in the social, financial, and work arena. Occurring at any time in a patient's life, cancer will likely alter the aspirations and direction of the individual. Treatment often involves a great deal of time off for evaluations, testing, treatment and the sequelae of that treatment. Return to work issues will depend on the type and extent of the cancer, its prognosis, and the likelihood of disease recurrence. Treatment is of different types and accompanying side effects. Treatment duration is unique to the individual, as are its anticipated debility and time of recovery. When formulating whether a patient will have to take a leave of absence, whether temporary or permanent, a clinician must take into account a number of variables. What are the physical, cognitive, communicative requirements, and job responsibilities of a patient? Will a patient's occupation or work environment have to change? Is it reasonable to expect that the patient can relearn a new job or profession? Can the patient do the new position without encountering new stressors and/or direct or indirect discrimination? More importantly, will the new position lead to possible injury for the patient or others working with him? Will the employer be able to reasonably accommodate the patient? Where a return to work is likely arduous for both the patient and the employer, the physiatrist must advocate for the patient and often educate treating physicians, the employer, disability carrier, and federal government.

Epidemiology

■ Cancer is the leading cause of long-term disability in the United States.
■ The most frequent cancer types associated with disability include breast, colon, and prostate.
■ The National Institutes of Health (NIH) estimated inclusive costs for treatment, lost productivity due to illness, and premature death at $201 billion in 2008.

■ UNUM, one of the largest disability insurance providers, estimated that 12% of its claims were related to cancer.

Etiology

■ Cancer care often requires a multitiered approach. It is taxing to the patient. Fear, concern, and worry are usually commonly shared, straining marital and family/friend relationships. A patient's treatment will constrain financial resources—personal, hospitals/clinics, insurance companies, and state and federal government agencies (Medicare, Medicaid).
■ Cancer often cannot be cured. It can go into remission. Its tendency to recur and metastasize requires close follow-up care.
■ When disease can be put into a cure or remission status, a patient may "initially" appear capable of returning to work. The individual wants to and he/she may appear seemingly "fine." There are necessary points of consideration:
  – Is the patient cognitively able to resume work? Neuropsychology and speech pathology evaluations of executive decision making, procedural detail, sequencing tasks, communication fluency, and carryover memory are crucial. Chemotherapy has many neurologic implications. Many cancers may later metastasize to the brain (e.g., lung, breast, thyroid, germ cell/reproductive tumors, and gastrointestinal tract).
  – In the treatment of both solid and liquid tumors there may be ongoing symptoms of pain and fatigue, which could contribute to performance difficulties and safety issues for both the employee as well as the employer.
  – Although the treatment of a cancer may be seemingly successful, the treatment may induce its own sequelae/impairment.
    • Mastectomy and axillary lymph node dissection: May lead to lymphedema, constraints in range of motion of an arm and shoulder joint with increased susceptibility to cellulitis. A patient may have acquired a neuropathy/neuropathic pain due to surgery (intercostobrachial cutaneous neuropathy) or chemotherapy (taxol, platins).

- Rectal cancer: radiation-induced proctitis, anal stenosis, and difficulties with defecation
- Involvement of the central nervous system by metastases/leptomeningeal disease can lead rapidly to encephalopathy, seizure, delirium, paraplegia, and neurogenic bowel/bladder.

Rehabilitation Implications

- An in-depth understanding of a patient's cancer is required.
- Education is critical. There needs to be coordination of information with the primary treating team; the physiatrist; and physical, occupational, and speech therapists. Often, wording used in reports is misleading or inaccurate. No evidence of disease refers only to no evidence of *detectable disease at that moment in time*. It does not necessarily mean cure.
- If future treatment (chemoradiation) or surgery is planned—a patient should be evaluated routinely by therapies in order to bolster range of motion, strength, gait, balance, proprioception, and endurance.
- If a patient's disease is stable (well managed and the patient tolerates treatment with minimal sequelae), one can consider a patient for return to work. This process is dependent on endurance. Pain and fatigue need to be under good control. Comprehension, insight, and task performance must approach premorbid levels.
- The physiatrist at this point coordinates a treatment plan with therapies. Routine follow-up will be critical in order to assess endurance and performance as the patient continues to be treated by the oncologist.

Helpful Hints

- The goal of rehabilitation medicine is to return a patient to the highest level of premorbid functioning.
- Many cancers follow an indolent pathway. Care is often complex, time consuming, and costly. Patients may experience treatment-induced fatigue, pain, cognitive dysfunction, and often impairments to mobility and self-care.
- Active disease in treatment often limits a patient's ability to return to work.

Suggested Readings

Alfano, CM, Ganz PA, Rowland JH, Hahn EE. Cancer survivorship and cancer rehabilitation: Revitalizing the link. *J Clin Oncol.* 2012;30:904–906.

Fu, J. The state of cancer rehabilitation. *J Palliative Care Med.* 2012;2:1–2.

Nontraditional Treatments: Acupuncture

Ying Guo MD MS

Description

Acupuncture, the insertion of sterile needles into acupuncture points of traditional meridians on the body, is a common and effective treatment for many symptoms in cancer patients.

Mechanism of Acupuncture

- Peripheral and central nervous system: Acupuncture increases endomorphin-1, beta endorphin, encephalin, and serotonin levels in plasma and brain tissue with effects on the autonomic nervous system.
- Endocrine system: hypothalamus
- Emotion: limbic system
- Fascia/connective tissue system: via a mechanotransduction-based mechanism; influences inflammation and immunity
- Muscular system: trigger-point treatment

Safety

- Minor adverse events estimated to be 14 per 10,000 sessions.
- Serious adverse events estimated to be 0.05 per 10,000 treatments ($5/10^6$).
- No significant bleeding side effects have been observed, even in patients with severe thrombocytopenia (20,000/mcL or lesser).
- Deep tissue acupuncture (i.e., more than 0.5 cm in depth) allowed if:
  - Absolute neutrophil count (ANC) is 1,000 or higher.
  - Platelet count is 50 K/mL or higher.
  - International normalized ratio (INR) is 1.5 or lower.
  - Patient is not taking anticoagulation medications.
- Cancer patients require certified practitioners who are experienced in treating patients with malignant diseases.

Evidence for Acupuncture Use

- Nausea/vomiting: National Institutes of Health (NIH) consensus: efficacious for chemotherapy nausea and vomiting
- Musculoskeletal symptoms in women on hormonal therapy for breast cancer
- Pain and xerostomia in patients following neck dissection and radiation-induced xerostomia.
- Fatigue

Payment

- Largely self-pay service; not yet covered by many insurance carriers and Medicare.

Helpful Hints

- PC 6 for nausea/vomiting
- LI 4 for headache
- LR 3 for anxiety
- Acupuncture software applications are available to locate these points. Acupressure (pressing on acupuncture points) can also be helpful.

Suggested Readings

Cabyoglu M, Ergene N, Tan U. The mechanism of acupuncture and clinical applications. *Int J Neurosci.* 2006;116(2):115–125.

Garcia MK, McQuade J, Haddad R. Systematic review of acupuncture in cancer care: A synthesis of the evidence. *J Clin Oncol.* 2013 Jan 22 [Epub ahead of print] PMID 23341529.

Lu W, Rosenthal DS. Acupuncture for cancer pain and related symptoms. *Curr Pain Headache Rep.* 2013;17(3):321.

Paley C. Acupuncture for the treatment of cancer pain: A systematic review. Response to authors. *Support Care Cancer.* 2013, Jan 11. [Epub ahead of print] PMID:23306936.

Nontraditional Treatments: Complementary, Alternative, and Integrative Medicine

Gabriel Lopez MD ▪ Carolina Gutierrez MD ▪ Richard Lee MD

Definition

Complementary and alternative medicine (CAM) is defined as a group of diverse medical and health care systems, practices, and products that are not normally considered to be conventional medicine. *Complementary medicine* refers to practices used alongside conventional medical therapies. *Alternative medicine* refers to practices used in place of conventional medical therapies. *Integrative medicine* describes a philosophy of practice using an evidence-based approach to merge conventional and nonconventional therapies.

Integrative Oncology

A comprehensive, personalized, evidence-based, and safe approach to merge conventional and complementary therapies in cancer care, taking into account patient psychosocial and physical well-being.

- Psychosocial well-being:
  - Stress-induced physiological changes may affect cancer development, treatment, and recurrence.
  - Provide support and education to patient, family, and caregivers
- Physical well-being:
  - Excess weight and physical inactivity contribute to increased incidence of numerous cancers.
  - Improved nutrition and increased physical activity can improve cancer treatment outcomes.
  - Appropriate referral to physical therapy and occupational therapy to optimize function during and after treatment

Prevalence

- 40% to 70% of cancer patients in the United States use CAM therapies.
- CAM use is higher among adults with functional limitations.
- Breast cancer patients have a more frequent use of CAM therapies than other cancer types.
- CAM use is higher among patients with advanced cancer.
- Cancer survivors are more likely to use CAM therapies than the general population.

Patient Motivations for Complementary and Alternative Medicine Use

- Improve quality of life and prolong life
- Boost the immune system
- Relieve symptoms
- Prevent cancer recurrence
- Aid conventional medical treatment
- Recommendation from family or friend

Complementary and Alternative Medicine Categories

- Natural products:
  - Herbal medicine, vitamins, minerals, probiotics
- Mind and body medicine:
  - Meditation, yoga, acupuncture, Qigong, tai chi
- Manipulative and body-based practices:
  - Massage, spinal manipulation (chiropractic, physical therapy)
- Other CAM practices:
  - Whole medical systems (Ayurvedic, traditional Chinese, naturopathy)
  - Energy therapies (magnet therapy, Reiki).
  - Movement therapies (Feldenkrais method)

Communication

- Up to 60% of cancer patients use CAM therapies without informing their health care team.
- The majority of cancer patients are open to discussion regarding use of CAM therapies.
- It is the responsibility of the practitioner to ask patients about CAM use and explore motivations.
- CAM therapies should not be dismissed as this can harm patient–practitioner relationship.
- Interdisciplinary approach to integrating CAM modalities is most effective and safe.

Safety Concerns of Herbs, Vitamins, or Supplements

- Quality:
  - No strict quality control, potential for harmful contaminants

IV: Special Concerns

■ Metabolic:
- May interfere with drug metabolism, acting as inducers or inhibitors, decreasing efficacy or increasing toxicity.
  • St. John's wort is an inducer of cytochrome P450 3A4.
■ Organ toxicity:
- Potential for hepatic or renal toxicity
  • Green tea with case reports of hepatotoxicity
■ Bleeding risk:
- Certain products may interfere with platelet function.
- Risk increased when combined with anticoagulants or antiplatelet agents.
- Hold prior to surgical procedures
  • Garlic extract, Gingko biloba, and fish oil may increase bleeding risk.

Evidence-Based Complementary and Alternative Medicine Modalities
■ Acupuncture
- Indications:
  • Pain (i.e., joint, headache, low back)
  • Xerostomia
  • Hot flashes
  • Nausea
  • Neuropathy
- Safety:
  • Precaution with neutropenia or thrombocytopenia
  • Avoid in limb with or at risk for lymphedema
■ Massage
- Indications:
  • Pain
  • Mood disturbance (anxiety or depression)
  • Constipation
  • Lymphedema (manual lymphatic drainage)
- Safety:
  • Encourage use of licensed oncology massage therapist.
  • Adjust type and level of massage to maximize safety.
  • Use precaution with neutropenia, thrombocytopenia, or dysfunctional platelets, recent surgery or radiation, metastatic bone disease.

■ Mind–body
- Meditation, yoga, tai chi
- Indications:
  • Stress reduction
  • Mood disturbance (anxiety)
  • Quality-of-life improvement
  • Insomnia
- Safety:
  • Risk of falls, injury with movement-based practices (i.e., yoga, tai chi)
  • Patient with severe anxiety may not tolerate one-on-one or group settings.
■ Music therapy
- Indications:
  • Stress reduction
  • Mood disturbance
  • Quality of life
- Safety:
  • Generally safe, recommend using a licensed music therapist

Helpful Hints
■ Ask patients about CAM use during initial encounter to enhance communication and maximize patient safety.
■ Enlist expertise of CAM or integrative medicine specialist if unsure of safe and appropriate use of a CAM modality.

Evidence-Based Resources
Natural Medicines Comprehensive Database. http://www.naturaldatabase.com/
Natural Standard. http://www.naturalstandard.com/
NCI Office of Cancer Complementary and Alternative Medicine (OCCAM). http://www.cancer.gov/cam
NIH National Center for Complementary and Alternative Medicine. http://nccam.nih.gov/
University of Texas MD Anderson Cancer Center Complementary/Integrative Medicine Education Resources. http://www.mdanderson.org/CIMER

Suggested Readings
Eheman C, Henley SJ, Ballard-Barbash R, et al. Annual Report to the Nation on the status of cancer 1975–2008, featuring cancers associated with excess weight and lack of sufficient physical activity. *Cancer.* 2012;118(9):2338–2366.
Rock CL, Doyle C, Demark-Wahnefried W, et al. Nutrition and physical activity guidelines for cancer survivors. *CA Cancer J Clin.* 2012;62:242–274.

Nontraditional Treatments: Massage

Pamela Austin Sumler LMT NCTMB

Description

Oncology massage therapy is a health profession concerned with nurturing the body, mind, and spirit of those who are dealing with cancer, through the application of safe massage adaptation (The Society for Oncology Massage 2012). Oncology massage therapists have specialized training that provide them with the knowledge and skills to customize massage treatments, according to the patient's specific cancer and cancer treatment-related needs. Therapists also consider the client's preferences and desired outcome and modify massage and bodywork techniques on the basis of the basic need of human touch, to enhance function, promote relaxation, and increase well-being.

Massage therapy consists of over 80 different treatment modalities, not all appropriate for the cancer patient. Individual consideration should be made before implementing them. Some of the most common include Swedish, deep tissue, chair massage, sports massage, trigger point, Asian massage, cranial-sacral, and healing touch.

Prevalence of Use

■ Oncology massage is finding an increasing role in managing symptoms associated with cancer and cancer treatments.

Indications

Cancer and cancer treatment-related symptoms include:
■ Pain
■ Anxiety
■ Nausea
■ Fatigue

Contraindications

■ Platelet count of less than 20,000
■ Rhabdomyolysis
■ Severe arteriosclerosis
■ Symptoms of deep venous thrombosis (DVT)
■ Recent limb perfusion chemotherapy treatment
■ Anticoagulant, antithrombotic, and thrombolytic agents
■ Chemotherapy-induced cutaneous reactions
■ Fever
■ Open wounds
■ Radiation dermatitis
■ Risk for fracture
■ Risk for lymphedema
■ Thrombocytopenia
■ Thromboembolism

Oncology Massage Treatment

Clinical considerations

■ Adjustments and modifications of the massage treatment should be made to the site, massage pressure, and patient's position during treatment, as indicated by cancer presentation, treatment, and comorbid conditions.

Cancer presentation

■ Primary tumor site and metastatic involvement:
  – Soft tissue
  – Bone
  – Vital organ

Cancer treatment

■ Chemotherapy: Review blood counts, monitor for signs of infections, avoid IV (intravenous) lines, observe fall precautions before and after massage, monitor fatigue.
■ Immunotherapy: Monitor for signs of infection and fatigue, avoid IV lines, observe fall precautions.
■ Radiation therapy: Monitor for skin changes, fatigue.
■ Stem cell transplantation: Review blood counts, monitor for infection, skin changes, fall precautions, fatigue.
■ Surgery: Avoid fluid shifts to area of recent surgery; monitor for skin changes, infection, and fatigue; observe fall precautions.

Comorbid conditions

■ Anticoagulation
  – For patients on Coumadin/warfarin, internal normalized ratio (INR) should be considered to help determine safe massage pressure.
    • INR 1.5 to 2: patients can easily bruise
    • INR 2 to 3: modify massage therapy pressure to Walton Scale Level 1 to 2.
    • INR more than 3.5: modify massage therapy pressure to Walton Scale 1.
■ Bone metastases: avoid other than light pressure over known lesions.
■ Palpable medical devices: avoid any direct pressure.
■ Cellulitis: avoid any direct pressure on involved areas.

- Deep vein thrombosis and pulmonary embolism (PE):
  - In patients with PE, screening with Doppler ultrasound of the upper and lower extremities should be considered to rule out DVT prior to massage of the extremities.
  - Avoid massage of an extremity with known or suspected DVT.
- Diabetes: skin precautions
- Heart failure: avoid significant fluid shifts.
- Pregnancy: avoid direct abdominal pressure or significant fluid shifts.

Massage pressure

- Walton Scale of Massage Pressures: 5-part scale of massage pressures and soft tissue body work technique:
  - 1—light lotioning
  - 2—heavy lotioning
  - 3—medium pressure
  - 4—strong pressure
  - 5—deep pressure

Complications of treatment

Adverse events are rare, but can occur. Reported adverse events include:

- Fractures
- Bruising
- Internal hemorrhage
- Hepatic hematoma
- Dislodged DVT and consequential embolus

Helpful Hint

- Light touch to the uninvolved hands or feet is usually not contraindicated and can help relieve symptoms. In general, avoid deep tissue massage in the cancer patient.

Suggested Reading

Collinge W, MacDonald G, Walton T. Massage in supportive cancer care. *Semin Oncol Nurs.* 2012 Feb;28(1):45–54.

Prognostication

David Hui MD MSc FRCPC

Importance of Communicating an Accurate Prognosis

- Affects personal decisions such as finances, functional goals, and life goals
- Influences health decisions
- Gives patients enough time to say "goodbye" to family and friends
- Respects patient autonomy
- Guides clinical decisions, such as initiation of chemotherapy and hospice referral.
- Approximately 90% of cancer patients would like to know about their prognosis.

Overview

- Prognostication consists of foreseeing (estimating the survival) and foretelling (breaking bad news):
  - Foreseeing requires a good understanding of the natural history of cancer (stage, treatment options), prognostic factors, and comorbidities.
    - Clinician prediction of survival involves an intuitive guess of patients' survival. Although this method often incorporates various prognostic factors, it is subjective and clinicians consistently overestimate survival.
    - Actuarial estimation of survival involves using prognostic factors and prognostic models to calculate life expectancy.
  - Foretelling involves understanding the patient's level of comprehension and emotional resilience, and delivering the information in a clear, empathic, and practical manner.
- Prognostication is a process that involves longitudinal evaluations and discussions tailored to patients' changing health status.

Median Survival for Common Advanced Cancers

- Lung cancer: stage IIIA 14 months, stage IIIB 10 months, stage IV 6 to 8 months
- Breast cancer: stage IV 22 to 24 months
- Colorectal cancer: stage IV 24 to 28 months
- Prostate cancer: stage IV 24 to 28 months
- Pancreatic cancer: stage III 8 to 9 months, stage IV 4 to 6 months

Prognostic Factors for Early-Stage Cancer: Stages I and II

- Cancer stage
- Cancer histology (e.g., grade, lymphovascular invasion)
- Genetic mutations and expression (e.g., p53, k-ras)

Prognostic Models for Early Stage Cancer

- Adjuvant online (www.adjuvantonline.com) is a useful website that provides survival data for breast, colon, and lung cancer, adjusted for various prognostic factors and treatment options.

Prognostic Factors for Advanced Cancer: Stages III and IV, Refractory or Recurrent Disease

- Debility (decreased performance status)
- Delirium
- Dyspnea
- Dysphagia–anorexia–cachexia
- Elevated C-reactive protein
- Leukocytosis
- Lymphocytopenia

Prognostic Models for Advanced Cancer

- The palliative prognostic score (PaP score) consists of six variables, including dyspnea, anorexia, Karnofsky performance status, clinician prediction of survival, total white blood cell count, and lymphocyte percentage.
- The palliative prognostic index consists of five variables, including the palliative performance scale, oral intake, edema, dyspnea at rest, and delirium.

Foretelling

- Setting—talk to the patient sitting down, ideally with family present (after asking for permission).
- Perception—explore what patients understand about their illness.
- Information—understand how the information can be useful to the patient.
- Knowledge—provide the prognostic information. Generally, specific numbers (i.e., 6 months) should

be avoided. Instead, use general terms such as "days," "weeks," "months," "years," and "decades."
■ Emotions—empathic comments can be useful.
■ Strategy—prognostic discussion often naturally leads to advance care planning and hospice discussions. It is important to communicate nonabandonment and provide the appropriate follow-up and referral (e.g., social work, counseling).

When to Share Prognosis?
■ When the patient (or family member) asks, "How long do I have?"
■ At initial oncology consultation
■ When expected survival is likely in terms of months
■ When the patient experiences a significant change in condition with a revised prognosis
■ When important clinical decisions such as palliative chemotherapy and hospice referral need to be made

Helpful Hints
■ Studies suggest that patients' level of hope does not decrease after hearing their prognosis.
■ It is important to avoid giving an exact number (expiration date) when sharing prognosis.

■ As patients get sicker, their desire for prognostic information decreases, whereas their families' need for information increases.
■ If a patient refuses to hear the prognosis, it may be important to ask for permission to discuss this information with caregivers to facilitate care planning.

Suggested Readings

Clayton JM, Butow PN, Arnold RM, Tattersall MH. Fostering coping and nurturing hope when discussing the future with terminally ill cancer patients and their caregivers. *Cancer.* 2005;103(9):1965–1975.

Glare PA, Sinclair CT. Palliative medicine review: Prognostication. *J Palliat Med.* 2008;11(1):84–103.

Hui D, Kilgore K, Nguyen L, et al. The accuracy of probabilistic versus temporal clinician prediction of survival for patients with advanced cancer: A preliminary report. *Oncologist.* 2011;16(11): 1642–1648.

Maltoni M, Caraceni A, Brunelli C, et al. Prognostic factors in advanced cancer patients: Evidence-based clinical recommendations—a study by the Steering Committee of the European Association for Palliative Care. *J Clin Oncol.* 2005;23(25):6240–6248.

Stone PC, Lund S. Predicting prognosis in patients with advanced cancer. *Ann Oncol.* 2007;18(6):971–976.

Rehabilitation Chaplain

J. Anthony Leachman MA BCC

Chaplaincy Care Pathway: for Rehabilitation Medicine Patients and Families

Adequately addressing the pastoral and emotional needs of cancer patients is frequently required for their successful rehabilitation. There can be a number of reasons for staff to refer for chaplaincy assessment and intervention (see Table 65.1).

Pathway Trigger for Chaplain Referral

- Trigger #1:
  - Cancer diagnosis is still recent or there is an exacerbation of symptoms.
  - Need to go back to primary service (i.e., back to leukemia service for treatment of infection/fever).
  - Patient and/or family are still overwhelmed, angry, fearful, crying.
- Trigger # 2:
  - Patient seems stuck or unable to move forward emotionally, owing to dwelling on cancer diagnosis or physical changes related to cancer treatments.
  - Lack of motivation or ability to find meaning in current circumstances
  - Noncompliance with treatment
  - Flat affect
  - Family or friends report patient is "giving up."
  - Comments made to family like, "Why did you/we let them do this surgery, treatment? Look at me."
- Trigger # 3:
  - Apparent need for narrative, a need to tell his or her story related to the cancer journey, to talk things out, to have someone demonstrate understanding of what the patient and/or family has been through and their related feelings.
  - Need for catharsis related to cancer experiences.
- Trigger # 4:
  - The 65+ age group (a common need to feel connected, and to share life experiences)
  - Women who are 65+ also desire a sense of self-transcendence
  - For the African American woman who has been the family leader, faith connects her to the traditions of her elders and is where she draws her personal strength in all her struggles/challenges, including cancer.

General Triggers for Chaplain Referral for Cancer and Noncancer Patients and/or Families

- Anxiety/fear/ineffective coping:
  - Subjective presentation:
    - Reports feeling blue, sad, or afraid
  - Objective presentation:
    - Patient is withdrawn, flat affect, poor concentration, few to no visitors.
- Emotional/spiritual distress
  - Subjective presentation:
    - "I'm starting to doubt God."
    - "Why is God letting this happen?"
  - Objective presentation:
    - Few to no visitors, frequently tearful
- Significant change in diagnosis/prognosis/condition
- Spiritual/religious needs (communion, prayer, etc.)
  - Subjective presentation:
    - Requests chaplain, minister, or priest
    - Requests prayer
- Diverse spiritual/cultural needs:
  - Subjective presentation:
    - Requesting a particular type of food (i.e., kosher) is an insight that religion or culture might have a significant meaning.
  - Objective presentation:
    - Symbols of religious meaning in room, such as the Koran, Bible, cross
- End-of-life concerns:
  - Subjective presentation:
    - Person expresses feelings of grief, denial, anger, bargaining, depression.
- Objective presentation:
  - Patient is tearful or cries frequently, yells at staff or is noncompliant, is withdrawn or shows symptoms of depression.
- Ethical issues:
  - Subjective presentation:
    - Verbalizing feelings of regret related to outcomes of disease or decisions made for treatment of disease
  - Objective presentation:
    - Disease process requires physician to discuss with family the need to consider a do-not-resuscitate (DNR) order and/or the need to withdraw more aggressive or curative means of treatment.

Table 65.1   Cancer Chaplaincy Issues, Interventions, and Desired Outcomes

Possible spiritual and/or emotional issues	Possible chaplain actions/interventions	Desired outcomes
• Disruption concern – Disruption in jobs or relationships: Often the cancer indicates the end of a career or will change means of job performance – Grief over loss of old way of life – New sense of calling (possibly bargaining—citing grief model) • Discomfort concern – Particularly in chronic pain and/or experience of suffering related to cancer and cancer treatment: "Why doesn't God just take him/her/me?" • Disfigurement concern • Concern about body image related to cancer: scarring, open wounds, deformities, amputation • Disability concern – Loss of function and independence related to cancer • Concerns about death with cancer diagnosis – Issues related to demands of rehab with a terminal diagnosis – Integrity versus despair issues—issues of fulfillment (Erikson) • Sense of blessing related to successes in cancer treatment and/or rehab process	• Ministry of narrative: Facilitating the telling of personal histories and experiences and their meaning to the patient, along with recent experiences/feelings related to the cancer process • Validation of patient and family experiences and feelings • Facilitate expressions of grief • Provide empathic, pastoral, and supportive presence • Silent, supportive presence • Facilitate expressions of feelings of anger, confusion, frustration • Explore issues of theodicy, providence, and meaning • Encourage family, cultural, and/or ecclesial support • Encourage self-care • Discuss resilience indicators • Help facilitate sacraments and rituals (rites) that meet patient emotional and spiritual needs • Prayer and supportive presence • Celebrate positive outcomes and/or the opportunity to go home with patient and family	• Patient will have an opportunity for catharsis • Patient will verbalize concerns and fears related to disruption • Patient will name personal strengths and resources to assist with coping • Patient will express a sense of connection/support in faith community and/or family • Patient will express anger/hurt • Patient will begin to form a new/hopeful future story • Patient will talk about experiences and beliefs that help give hope • Patient will verbalize body image concerns and progress to new self-image and personal integrity • Patient will discuss and identify spiritual resources • Patient will explore meaning he has found in his experiences • Patient will discuss meaning of death • Patient will have opportunities to express gratitude for blessing • Patient and family will have opportunity to give thanks in a way that is meaningful to them

Acknowledgments

- Credit and gratitude are due to Susan Nance, ACPE ThM, who developed the template for this pathway based on Sue Wintz's document concerning spiritual pathways; and Memorial Hermann in their use and validation of the effectiveness of the Chaplaincy Pathway.
- Credit and gratitude are due to Brent Peery, D. Minn, BCC, for his development of Memorial Hermann's Chaplaincy Charting Model, and his focus on Outcome-Based Chaplaincy, which also influenced this document.

Suggested Readings

Bean KB, Wagner K. Self-transcendence, illness distress, and quality of life among liver transplant recipients. *J Theory Construction and Testing.* 2006;10(2).

Billman, KD, Migliore DL. *Rachel's Cry.* Eugene, OR: Wipf & Stock Publishers; 1999. (The authors make reference to the "womanist" as the African American woman who was the leader in her home, her example of strength and its source.)

Boswell B, Hamer M, Knight S, et al. Dance of disability and spirituality. *J Rehab,* 2007;73(4):33–40.

Carpenito LJ. *Nursing Diagnosis—Application and Clinical Practice.* 2nd ed. Philadelphia: J.B. Lippincott Company; 1987.

Erikson, EH. *Identity and the Life Cycle.* New York, NY: W. W. Norton; 1980.

Frankl, VE. *Man's Search for Meaning.* Boston, MA: Beacon Press; 2006.

The Joanna Briggs Institute. The Joanna Briggs Institute for Best Practice Information Sheet: The psychosocial and spiritual experiences of elderly individuals recovering from a stroke. *Nurs Health Sci.* 2010;12:515–518

Lester AD. *Hope in Pastoral Care and Counseling.* Louisville, KY: Westminster John Knox Press; 1995.

Lewis JM. Pastoral Assessment in Hospital Ministry, A Conversational Approach. *Chaplaincy Today,* 2002;18(2). Chaplain Lewis' assessment outline seems particularly useful in rehab patients. I changed the word "crisis" to "concern" due to colleagues having difficulty with the use of "crisis" with the absence of significant emotional responses.

Nance S, Ramsey K, Leachman JA. Chaplaincy care pathways and clinical pastoral education. *J Pastoral Care Counsel.* 2009; July.

Waldron-Perrine B, Rapport L, Hanks R, et al. Religion and spirituality in rehabilitation outcomes among individuals with traumatic brain injury. *Rehab Psychol.* 2011;56(2):107–116.

White B, Driver S, Warren AM. Resilience and indicators of adjustment during rehabilitation from a spinal cord injury. *Rehab Psychol,* 2010 February;55(1):23–32.

Wintz S. Spiritual pathways in the nursery ICU. *Oates* 2003;6.

Rehabilitation at the End of Life

Ki Y. Shin MD

Palliative Medicine
- The management of patients with progressive and advanced disease in which prognosis is limited and the focus of care is on quality of life and the relief of suffering.

World Health Organization Cancer Pain and Palliative Care Report
- Fundamental principles of palliative care:
  - Affirm life and regard dying as a normal process.
  - Neither hasten nor postpone death.
  - Provide relief from pain and other distressing symptoms.
  - Integrate the psychological and spiritual aspects of patient care.
  - Offer a support system to help patients live as actively as possible until death.
  - Offer a support system to help family members cope during the patient's illness and their bereavement.

Rehabilitation Medicine and Palliative Care: Similarities
- Both aim to support qualify of life and to relieve discomfort.
- Framework for intervention is similar with a multidisciplinary team working together to adequately assess and treat the patient.
- Emphasis is not necessarily on the disease process, but on physical symptoms, limitations of the patient, and how to improve or relieve them.
- Importance of including the family in patient care and providing family support and education.

Rehabilitation Medicine and Palliation Difference
- Palliative care focuses on symptom control. Rehabilitation at the end of life also focuses on maintaining quality of life through functional activities.

Importance of Appropriate Goal Setting
- Improving function and preserving patient autonomy and safety are still the rehabilitation goals.

- In the face of medical and functional decline, the patient and family need to be informed and aware of the disease status and prognosis.
- As Cheville reminds us, "Are the treatment goals humane and ethical in the unique context of each patient's cancer, and do they reflect the patient's wishes?"
- With the urgency of limited patient time and energy and to maximize patient buy-in, it is important to have the patient take an active role in rehabilitation goal setting. "What do you want to be able to do and why?"

Rehabilitation Interventions
- Transfer, wheelchair, and gait training
- Activities of daily living (ADLs) training
- Positioning and pressure relief techniques
- Chest physiotherapy
- Swallowing assessment and exercises to improve dysphagia
- Edema management
- Physical modalities to treat pain
- Bracing and splinting to relieve pain and assist with mobility
- Caregiver training

Caregiver Issues
- Concerns:
  - Fear of hurting the patient physically by moving him or her
  - Fear of hurting oneself when moving or transferring the patient
  - Lack of clarity regarding how hard to push patient
- Family education in transfer training and positioning can decrease the perceived stress of providing care and also the patient's concern about being a burden.

Depression
- When active rehabilitation ceases, hope can frequently be lost.
- Can limit participation in therapies
- Pharmacologic intervention and counseling can assist
- Psychoactive stimulants, such as methylphenidate, may be used to increase patient alertness and assist with active participation.

Disposition Planning

- As the patient's disease progresses, decline in function may be significant and the resources may not be available for care at home.
- The rehabilitation team can assist with recommendations for placement in assisted living, skilled nursing facility, nursing home, or hospice as appropriate.

Symptom Control

- Once a safe discharge setting has been addressed, rehabilitation at the very end of life becomes primarily an issue of symptom control.
- Pharmacologic management of distressing symptoms including pain, dyspnea, agitation, delirium, and respiratory secretions may be needed with the assistance from palliative care specialists as available.

Helpful Hints

- Palliative care and rehabilitation medicine have similarities in terms of goals and methods.
- End-of-life rehabilitation may be just as important as restorative rehabilitation in terms of patient and family sense of urgency and appreciation.
- Appropriate patient, family, rehabilitation team, and oncology team goals can make the transition to palliative care an easier one. This is accomplished best with frequent communication among the patient, family, and medical teams.

Suggested Readings

Cheville A. Rehabilitation of patients with advanced cancer. *Cancer.* 2001;92:1039–1048.

Mackey KC, Sparling JW. Experiences of older women with cancer receiving hospice care: Significance for physical therapy. *Phys Ther.* 2000;80:459–468.

Yoshioka H. Rehabilitation for the terminal cancer patient. *Am J Phys Med Rehabil.* 1994;73:199–206.